Lunch ! 2022 Recipe Book

100 Delicious and Healthy Recipes to Replace Processed Food Ingredients

Judy R. Miller

Contents

Chapter One

SANDWICHES WITH SLOW-COOKED CORNED BEEF

1 5 servings | 15 minutes of prep time | 4 hours and 15 minutes of cooking time | 4 hours and 15 minutes of total time FACTS ABOUT THE NUTRITION

229 calories | 4.2 grams of carbs | 15.1 grams of fat | 15 grams of protein | 78 milligrams of cholesterol

INGREDIENTS

2 corned beef briskets (3 pounds each) with spice packets

peppercorns (about 1/4 cup)

2 beer bottles (12 fluid ounces)

1 garlic bulb, peeled and divided cloves

2 leaves of bay

DIRECTIONS

Fill a big saucepan halfway with corned beef briskets. One of the spice packets should be used, while the other should be discarded or saved for later. Pour in the beer and cover the briskets with 1 inch of water. Bay leaves, peppercorns, and garlic cloves should all be added at this point. Bring to a boil, uncovered.

Reduce the heat to medium-low and simmer for 4 to 5 hours, monitoring regularly and adding additional water as needed to keep the meat covered.

Remove the meat from the saucepan with caution, as it will be very delicate. Allow to rest for 10 minutes on a chopping board. Serve by slicing or shredding. The cooking liquid is discarded, but it may be saved and used to prepare cabbage and other vegetables.

QUINOA SALAD FROM THE MEDITERRANEAN

8 servings | 15 minutes of prep time | 20 minutes of cooking time | 35 minutes total FACTS ABOUT THE NUTRITION

278 calories | 20.1 grams of carbs | 13.9 grams of fat | 18.4 grams of protein | 45 milligrams of cholesterol

INGREDIENTS

2 cubes chicken bouillon 2 cups water 1/2 cup crumbled feta cheese

fresh parsley, chopped

1 garlic clove (crushed)

fresh chives, chopped

1 quinoa cup (raw)

salt, 1/2 teaspoon

2 big cooked chicken breasts, peeled and chopped into bite-size pieces

lemon juice, 2/3 cup

1 medium sliced red onion

balsamic vinegar, 1 tblsp

1 pound chopped green bell pepper

olive oil, 1/4 cup

kalamata olives (chopped) 1/2 cup

DIRECTIONS

In a saucepan, combine the water, bouillon cubes, and garlic. Reduce the heat to medium-low, cover, and cook for 15 to 20 minutes, or until the quinoa is cooked and the liquid has been absorbed. Scrape the quinoa into a large basin and discard the garlic clove.

In a small bowl, combine the quinoa, chicken, onion, bell pepper, olives, feta cheese, parsley, chives, and salt. Lemon juice, balsamic vinegar, and olive oil should be drizzled over the salad. Stir everything together until everything is uniformly distributed. Serve hot or cold, depending on your preference.

BEEF STEW OF KYLE'S CHOICE

10 servings | 30 minutes of prep time | 7 hours 15 minutes of cooking time | 7 hours 45 minutes of total time FACTS ABOUT THE NUTRITION

617 calories | 46.6 grams of carbs | 34.3 grams of fat | 30.7 grams of protein | 100 milligrams of cholesterol

INGREDIENTS

2 cups boiling water 3 pounds beef stew meat cubed

1 tablespoon flour, all-purpose

onion soup mix, 2 (1 ounce) envelopes

salt, 1/2 teaspoon

butter, 3 tablespoons

olive oil, 3 tablespoons

3 quartered big onions

3 TBS WORCESTERSHIRE

2 tbsp. garlic (minced)

peeled and cut into 2-inch pieces 1 pound carrots

burgundy wine (half a cup)

2 (6 ounce) fresh button mushrooms, halved 4 big potatoes, cubed

1 tsp parsley powder

a quarter cup of warm water

1 1/2 tsp. black pepper, freshly ground

cornstarch, 3 tblsp

DIRECTIONS

In a sealable bag, toss the beef with the flour and salt until well covered.

Over medium-high heat, heat the oil in a large pan. In a pan, combine the beef and Worcestershire sauce; heat until the meat is equally browned on all sides; transfer to a slow cooker, but leave the skillet untouched. In the slow cooker, combine the carrots, potatoes, parsley, and pepper.

In a small dish, combine the hot water with the soup mix; pour into the slow cooker.

Over medium-high heat, melt the butter in the skillet. Return the pan to the heat and sauté the onion and garlic in the melted butter until tender. Transfer the onion and garlic to the slow cooker and return the skillet to the heat. In a pan, combine the wine and mushrooms; heat until the mushrooms have absorbed the wine; transfer to a slow cooker.

Cook for one hour on High with the lid on the slow cooker. Reduce to low heat and simmer for 6 to 8 hours, or until the meat is fork-tender. Warm the water and cornstarch together, then whisk it into the stew. Cook, uncovered, for 15 minutes or until the stew thickens.

SALAD WITH THAI CUCUMBER

4 servings | 15 minutes to prepare | 30 minutes to cook

FACTS ABOUT THE NUTRITION

238 calories | 37.1 grams of carbs | 9.4 grams of fat | 5.8 grams of protein | 0 milligrams of cholesterol

INGREDIENTS

3 big cucumbers, peeled, half lengthwise, seeded, and thinly sliced

2 seeded and sliced jalapeo peppers

1 tsp sodium

cilantro, chopped

white sugar, 1/2 cup

1 pound peanuts, chopped

rice wine vinegar (half cup)

DIRECTIONS

In a strainer, toss the cucumbers with the salt and drain for 30 minutes in the sink. Drain and wipe dry with paper towels after rinsing in cold water.

In a mixing dish, combine the sugar and vinegar and whisk to dissolve the sugar. Toss together the cucumbers, jalapeo peppers, and cilantro. Before serving, streusel with chopped peanuts.

TOMATO SANDWICH AT ITS BEST

2 people | 10 minutes to prepare | 5 minutes to cook | 15 minutes total FACTS ABOUT THE NUTRITION

509 calories | 43.2 grams of carbs | 34.8 grams of fat | 9.6 grams of protein | 14 milligrams of cholesterol

INGREDIENTS

olive oil, 2 tablespoons

1 tsp. oregano (dried)

balsamic vinegar, 2 teaspoons

black pepper, 1/4 teaspoon

3 tablespoons grated cheese 4 ripe tomatoes halved parmesan cheese

mayonnaise, 3 tblsp.

4 gently toasted bread slices

1 tsp parsley, dry

DIRECTIONS

Preheat the oven to broiling temperature.

Combine the olive oil and vinegar in a small mixing basin. Toss the tomatoes in the mixture and let them marinate for a few minutes, swirling periodically.

Meanwhile, mix mayonnaise, parsley, oregano, black pepper, and 4 tablespoons Parmesan cheese together in a small bowl. Each piece of toasted bread should be topped with the mixture. Top 2 slices with marinated tomatoes and the remaining Parmesan cheese.

Broil for 5 minutes, or until the cheese is golden brown, on a baking sheet. Open-faced or closed-faced, serve immediately.

GOAT CHEESE BEET SALAD

6 people | 10 minutes to prepare | 30 minutes to cook | 40 minutes total 347 calories | 25 grams of carbohydrates | 26.1 grams of fat | 5.3 grams of protein | 7 milligrams of cholesterol

INGREDIENTS

4 medium beets, washed, trimmed, and half-cut

1/2 cup concentrated frozen orange juice

walnuts, 1/3 cup

balsamic vinegar (quarter cup)

maple syrup, 3 tbsp

1/2 cup olive oil (extra virgin)

1 mixed baby salad greens (10 oz.) package

goat cheese (2 oz.)

DIRECTIONS

Pour enough water to cover the beets in a saucepan. Bring to a boil, then reduce to a low heat and simmer for 20 to 30 minutes, or until the potatoes are cooked. Cut into cubes after draining and cooling.

Put the walnuts in a pan over medium-low heat while the beets are cooking. Stir in the maple syrup after the mixture is heated and beginning to toast. Remove from the fire and put aside to cool. Cook and whisk until evenly coated.

To create the dressing, combine orange juice concentrate, balsamic vinegar, and olive oil in a small bowl.

Place a big handful of baby greens on each of four salad dishes, then evenly distribute candied walnuts on top. Over the greens, scatter equal quantities of beets and dabs of goat cheese. Using some of the dressing, drizzle it over each dish.

SALAD WITH QUINOA AND CRANBERRY

6 Servings | 10 minutes to prepare | 20 minutes to cook | 2 hours and 30 minutes total Calories: 176 | Carbohydrates: 31.6g | Fat: 3.9g | Protein: 5.4g | Cholesterol: 0mg NUTRITION FACTS Calories: 176 | Carbohydrates: 31.6g | Fat: 3.9g | Protein: 5.4g

INGREDIENTS

1/4 cup minced fresh cilantro 1 1/2 cups water

1 lime, juiced 1 cup uncooked quinoa

1/4 cup sliced toasted almonds 1/4 cup red bell pepper, diced

1/2 cup minced carrots 1/4 cup yellow bell pepper, chopped

1 finely sliced red onion (small)

cranberries (dried) 1/2 cup

1 tblsp curry powder

To taste, season with salt and black pepper.

DIRECTIONS

Fill a pot halfway with water and cover. Bring to a boil over high heat, then add the quinoa, cover, and continue to cook on low heat for 15 to 20 minutes, or until all of the water has been absorbed. Scrape the mixture into a mixing dish and refrigerate until cool.

Stir in the red and yellow bell peppers, red onion, curry powder, cilantro, lime juice, sliced almonds, carrots, and cranberries after the sauce has cooled. Add salt and pepper to taste. Serve chilled.

SANDWICH CUBAN FOR MIDNIGHT

4 servings | 20 minutes to prepare | 5 minutes to cook FACTS ABOUT THE NUTRITION

1096 calories | 44.1 grams of carbs | 84.4 grams of fat | 43.3 grams of protein | 127 milligrams of cholesterol

INGREDIENTS

mayonnaise, 1 cup

5 tablespoons Italian dressing 1/2 pound cooked thinly sliced ham

1/2 pound of cheese

4 lengthwise-split hoagie rolls

1 cup slices of dill pickle

4 tsp mustard (prepared)

olive oil (1/2 cup)

deli turkey flesh, thinly sliced

DIRECTIONS

Mayonnaise and Italian dressing are combined in a small bowl. On hoagie rolls, spread the mixture. Make a mustard smear on each roll. Arrange turkey, ham, and cheese in layers on each bun. Dill pickle slices go on top of each. Brush tops and bottoms of sandwiches with olive oil before closing them.

Over medium high heat, heat a nonstick skillet. In a skillet, place sandwiches. Cook for 2 minutes on a dish covered in aluminum foil, pushing down on the sandwiches. Cook for 2 minutes longer, or until cheese is melted on the other side. Remove from heat, transfer to plates, and cut diagonally in half.

MUSHROOM SOUP WITH A CREAMY FLAVOR

6 servings | 15 minutes of prep time | 1 hour and 20 minutes of cooking time | 1 hour and 35 minutes of total time FACTS ABOUT THE NUTRITION

272 calories | 12.2 grams of carbs | 23.3 grams of fat | 6.9 grams of protein | 78 milligrams of cholesterol

INGREDIENTS

1 tbsp. butter (unsalted)

2 pounds fresh mushrooms, cut 2 garlic cloves, peeled

1 teaspoon salt 1 cup water 4 cups chicken broth

1 finely chopped yellow onion

1 quart heavy cream (whipped)

1 1/2 tbsp flour (all-purpose)

1 tsp salt, freshly ground black pepper, to taste

fresh thyme (6 sprigs)

1 teaspoon fresh thyme leaves (to taste) as a garnish

DIRECTIONS

In a large soup pot, melt the butter over medium-high heat; sauté the mushrooms in the butter with 1 pinch of salt until they release their juices; decrease heat to low. Cook, turning often, until the mushrooms are golden brown and the fluids have evaporated, approximately 15 minutes. If wanted, save aside a few pretty mushroom pieces to use as garnish later. Cook for a another 5 minutes, or until the onion is tender and transparent.

To get rid of the raw flour flavor, sprinkle flour into the mushroom mixture and simmer for 2 minutes, stirring constantly. Add thyme sprigs and garlic cloves to mushroom mixture in a tiny bundle tied with kitchen twine. In a mixing bowl, combine the chicken stock and water. Cook for 1 hour after bringing to a simmer. The thyme bundle should be removed.

In small batches, purée the soup in a high-powered blender until smooth and thick.

Stir in the cream and return the soup to the stove. Season to taste with salt and pepper, then serve in dishes with the saved mushroom slices and a few thyme leaves.

CHICKEN IN A SLOW COOKER

8 servings | 5 minutes to prepare | 6:35 minutes to cook

FACTS ABOUT THE NUTRITION

589 calories | 90 grams of carbs | 9.5 grams of fat | 34.2 grams of protein | 59 milligrams of cholesterol

INGREDIENTS

4 big chicken breast halves, skinless and boneless

Worcestershire sauce, 2 tblsp.

ketchup (around a cup)

chili powder (1/2 teaspoon)

mustard 2 tbsp

cayenne pepper (1/8 teaspoon)

lemon juice (2 teaspoons)

2 tblsp. spicy pepper sauce (or to taste) (optional)

garlic powder, 1/4 teaspoon

Split into 8 sandwich rolls

maple syrup, 1/2 gallon

DIRECTIONS

In the bottom of a slow cooker, arrange the chicken breasts. Combine the ketchup, mustard, lemon juice, garlic powder, maple syrup, Worcestershire sauce, chili powder, cayenne pepper, and hot sauce in a mixing bowl and whisk well to combine.

Cook for 6 hours on Low after pouring the sauce over the chicken. Cook for 30 minutes longer, shredding the chicken with two forks. Fill the sandwich buns with the chicken and sauce.

BORSCHT SOUP FROM UKRAINE

10 servings | 25 minutes to prepare | 40 minutes to cook | 1 hour and 15 minutes total FACTS ABOUT THE NUTRITION

257 calories | 24.4 grams of carbs | 13.8 grams of fat | 10.1 grams of protein | 31 milligrams of cholesterol

INGREDIENTS

1 pork sausage (16 oz.)

1 medium cabbage head, cored and shredded

peeled and shredded 3 medium beets

1 drained 8-ounce can of chopped tomatoes

3 shredded carrots (peeled)

3 medium peeled and diced baking potatoes salt and pepper to taste 3 garlic cloves, minced

1 tsp. oil

1 teaspoon white sugar, or to taste 1 big chopped onion 1/2 cup sour cream for sour cream topping 1 (6 ounce) can tomato paste

1 tbsp. fresh parsley (chopped) to serve as a garnish

water, 3/4 cup

DIRECTIONS

In a medium-high-heat skillet, crumble the sausage (if using). Cook, stirring constantly, until the sauce has thickened and is no longer pink. Turn off the heat and put the pan aside.

Bring 2 quarts of water to a boil in a big saucepan halfway filled with water. Cover the pot with the sausage. Raise the temperature to high and bring the water back to a boil. Cook until the beets have lost their color, around 10 minutes. Cook for 15 minutes or until the carrots and potatoes are soft. Combine the cabbage and diced tomatoes in a mixing bowl.

Over medium heat, heat the oil in a skillet. Cook until the onion is soft. In a large mixing bowl, combine the tomato paste and water until well combined. Fill the kettle halfway with water. Cover and remove from the fire after the raw garlic has been added. Allow for a 5-minute cooling period. Salt, pepper, and sugar to taste.

Serve with sour cream and fresh parsley, if preferred.

SALAD WITH DIVINE EGG

4 servings | 5 minutes to prepare | 16 minutes to cook FACTS ABOUT THE NUTRITION

212 calories | 3.2 grams of carbohydrate | 18.4 grams of fat | 9.9 grams of protein | 284 milligrams of cholesterol

INGREDIENTS

6 eggs are required.

1 lemon, freshly squeezed

mayonnaise (quarter cup)

green onions, chopped

salt and pepper to taste 1 teaspoon Dijon mustard

1 teaspoon yellow mustard (prepared)

DIRECTIONS

Cover the egg with cold water in a saucepan. Bring the water to a boil, then remove it from the heat right away. Allow 10 to 12 minutes for the eggs to sit in the boiling water covered. Remove from the boiling water and let it cool before peeling.

Put the eggs in an ice bath before peeling them to speed up the chilling process.

Mayonnaise, Dijon mustard, yellow mustard, lemon juice, and green onions should all be mixed together in a medium mixing basin. Prepare the eggs by chopping them into large bits and gently mixing them in with the dressing. Using salt and pepper, season to taste.

JELLY SANDWICH WITH GRILLED PEANUT BUTTER

1 serving | 5 minutes to prepare | 8 minutes to prepare | 13 minutes to cook 273 calories | 35.5 grams of carbohydrates | 12.5 grams of fat | 5.3 grams of protein | 22 milligrams of cholesterol

INGREDIENTS

butter, 2 tablespoons

1 tsp. pb

white bread, two pieces

2 tbsp. fruit jelly (any flavor)

DIRECTIONS

Preheat a griddle or a pan to 350°F (175 degrees C).

Each piece of bread should be butter-side down. One piece of bread should have peanut butter on the unbuttered side and jelly on the buttered side. On the griddle, place one slice with the greased side down. Place the second slice on top of the first, so that the peanut butter and jelly are in the center. Cook for 4 minutes per side on each side, or until golden brown and well cooked.

GARBANZOS AND ESPINACAS (SPINACH WITH GARBANZO BEANS)

4 servings | 15 minutes to prepare | 10 minutes to cook

FACTS ABOUT THE NUTRITION

169 calories | 26 grams of carbs | 4.9 grams of fat | 7.3 grams of protein | 0 milligrams of cholesterol

INGREDIENTS

1 tbsp olive oil extra-virgin

1 can drained garbanzo beans 4 chopped garlic cloves 1/2 teaspoon cumin

1/2 teaspoon salt 1 onion, chopped

1 (10-ounce) carton thawed and well-drained frozen chopped spinach

1. In a pan over medium-low heat, heat the olive oil. 5 minutes in the oil, cook the garlic and onion until transparent. Add the spinach, garbanzo beans, cumin, and salt, and stir to combine. As the mixture cooks, mash the beans softly with your stirring spoon. Cook until everything is hot.

Chapter Two

SALMON, ONION, AND TOMATO SALAD WITH MARINATED C UCUMBER

6 servings | 15 minutes to prepare | 2 hours to cook
Calories: 156 | Carbohydrates: 19.6g | Fat: 9.5g | Protein: 1.8g | Cholesterol: 0mg NUTRITION FACTS Calories: 156 | Carbohydrates: 19.6g | Fat: 9.5g | Protein: 1.8g

INGREDIENTS

1 quart of liquid

1 tbsp. black pepper, finely ground

12 cup white vinegar (distilled)

3 peeled and thinly sliced cucumbers Thickness: 1/4"

Vegetable oil, 1/4 cup

3 peeled and halved tomatoes

sugar, 1/4 cup

1 onion, cut into rings and sliced

salt, 2 tsp

DIRECTIONS

In a large mixing basin, whisk together the water, vinegar, oil, sugar, salt, and pepper until smooth; toss in the cucumbers, tomatoes, and onion.

Refrigerate for at least 2 hours, covered with plastic wrap.

ORZO WITH LEMON CHICKEN

12 servings | 20 minutes to prepare | 1 hour and 20 minutes to cook FACTS ABOUT THE NUTRITION

167 calories | 21.7 grams of carbs | 4.1 grams of fat | 12.1 grams of protein | 20 milligrams of cholesterol

INGREDIENTS

1 bay leaf 1 teaspoon olive oil 8 oz orzo pasta 1 bay leaf

3 cartons fat-free, low-sodium chicken broth (32 ounces) 3 carrots, diced, or to taste

lemon juice, 1/2 cup

1 lemon, zested 1 onion, diced 8 ounces 3 ribs celery, chopped 1 lemon, zested 2 garlic cloves, minced (cooked chicken breasts)

1 bag of baby spinach leaves (8 oz.)

1 tsp thyme (dried)

1 lemon, peeled and sliced to serve as a garnish (optional)

1 tsp. oregano (dried)

Parmesan cheese (grated): 1/4 cup (optional)

To taste, season with salt and black pepper.

DIRECTIONS

Bring a large pot of water to a boil, lightly salted. Cook orzo in boiling water for approximately 5 minutes, or until partly cooked but not soft; drain and rinse with cold water until totally cool.

In a big saucepan over medium heat, heat the olive oil. Cook and stir carrots, celery, and onion in heated oil for 5 to 7 minutes, or until the veggies soften and the onion becomes translucent. Cook and stir for 1 minute longer, or until garlic is fragrant. Season with thyme, oregano, salt, black pepper, and bay leaf, and simmer for another 30 seconds before adding the chicken broth.

Raise the temperature of the broth to high. Reduce heat to medium-low and simmer, partially covered, for approximately 10 minutes, or until the veggies are just tender.

In a large mixing bowl, combine the orzo, lemon juice, and lemon zest; add the chicken. Cook for approximately 5 minutes, or until the chicken and orzo are hot. Cook for 2 to 3 minutes, or until the baby spinach has wilted into the broth and the orzo is cooked. Serve the soup in dishes with lemon slices and grated Parmesan cheese on top.

SPROUTS OF PARMESAN BRUXELLES

2 servings | 10 minutes of prep time | 15 minutes of cooking time | 25 minutes total FACTS ABOUT THE NUTRITION

203 calories | 6.3 grams of carbs | 18.9 grams of fat | 4.2 grams of protein | 50 milligrams of cholesterol

INGREDIENTS

14 cup butter

14 cup butter

2 garlic cloves (minced)

2 tbsp. grated Parmesan cheese (or to taste)

14 cup butter

To taste, season with salt and black pepper.

trimmed and halved 6 Brussels sprouts

DIRECTIONS

3 minutes on medium heat, heat a frying pan until it is hot.
1 tablespoon butter, melted; garlic, cooked and stirred for 30 seconds or until fragrant. Cover and heat until golden brown, about 4 to 6 minutes, with 1 tablespoon butter and Brussels sprouts cut-side down.

1 tablespoon butter, 1 turn of Brussels sprouts Cook
for another 3 minutes, covered, until the opposite side is browned. Place on a platter to serve. Season with salt and black pepper and parmesan cheese.

WHITE RICE OF BRAZIL

8 servings | 15 minutes to prepare | 30 minutes to cook

FACTS ABOUT THE NUTRITION

201 calories | 37.5 grams of carbs | 3.7 grams of fat | 3.4 grams of protein | 0 milligrams of cholesterol

INGREDIENTS

2 c. white rice, long grain

2 tbsp. oil

2 tbsp. onion (minced)

1 tsp sodium

2 garlic cloves, chopped

4 cup of steaming water

DIRECTIONS

Rinse the rice completely in cold water in a colander and leave aside.

Over medium heat, heat the oil in a saucepan. For 1 minute, cook the onion in the oil. Cook until the garlic is golden brown, stirring occasionally. Cook and stir until the rice starts to brown, then add the rice and salt. Stir in a cup of boiling water to the rice mixture. Reduce the heat to low, cover the pot, and cook for 20 to 25 minutes, or until the water is absorbed.

SPICY APPLESAUCE FOR THE SLOW COOKER

8 servings | 10 minutes of prep time | 6 hours and 30 minutes of cooking time | 6 hours and 40 minutes of total time FACTS ABOUT THE NUTRITION

150 calories | 39.4 grams of carbs | 0.2 grams of fat | 0.4 grams of protein | 0 milligrams of cholesterol

INGREDIENTS

8 thinly sliced apples, peeled, cored

3/4 cup brown sugar, tightly packed

water (1/2 cup)

1 teaspoon pumpkin pie seasoning

DIRECTIONS 1. In a slow cooker, combine the apples and water; simmer for 6 to 8 hours on Low. Cook for a further 30 minutes after adding the brown sugar and pumpkin pie spice.

SALMON BURGERS WITH LEMON

6 people | 12 minutes to prepare | 8 minutes to cook | 20 minutes total FACTS ABOUT THE NUTRITION

209 calories | 5.3 grams of carbs | 11.4 grams of fat | 20.5 grams of protein | 97 milligrams of cholesterol

INGREDIENTS

1 drained and flaked salmon can (16 ounces)

1 tsp basil powder

2 quail

1 tsp. flakes de pimentón

fresh parsley, chopped

1 tsp. oil

2 tblsp onion, cut finely

2 TBS MAYONNAISE (LIGHT)

14 cup dried Italian bread crumbs, seasoned

lemon juice, 1 tbsp

lemon juice, 2 teaspoons

1 tsp basil powder

DIRECTIONS

Toss the salmon, eggs, parsley, onion, breadcrumbs, 2 tablespoons lemon juice, 1/2 teaspoon basil, and red pepper flakes together in a medium mixing bowl. Make 6 1/2-inch thick patties.

A big skillet with medium heat is used to heat the oil. Cook the patties in the heated oil for 4 minutes each side, or until beautifully browned.

Combine mayonnaise, 1 tablespoon lemon juice, and a sprinkle of basil in a small mixing dish. Serve with patties as a sauce.

FAJITA MELTS FROM CHICKEN

8 servings | 10 minutes of prep time | 25 minutes of cooking time | 35 minutes total FACTS ABOUT THE NUTRITION

397 calories | 19.9 grams of carbs | 16.6 grams of fat | 40.3 grams of protein | 104 milligrams of cholesterol

INGREDIENTS

3 tbsp. oil

taco seasoning blend, 2 tblsp

6 skinless, boneless chicken breast halves, thinly sliced 6 (6 ounce) skinless, boneless chicken breast halves

salsa (1 cup)

1/2 pound onions, sliced

8 slices of French bread (1/2 inch thick)

red bell pepper, sliced 1/2 cup

2 c. Cheddar cheese (shredded)

Tomato juice (1/2 cup)

DIRECTIONS

Over medium-high heat, heat the oil in a large pan. Cook for 5 minutes, stirring occasionally, until the chicken is lightly browned.

Cook and stir for 5 minutes, or until the veggies are soft, adding the sliced onions and red peppers last. Mix thoroughly after adding the tomato juice and taco spice. Cook for a further

7 minutes, or until the sauce has thickened and the chicken is well covered.

Preheat the broiler in the oven and place the oven rack approximately 6 inches away from the heat source.

Over each piece of French bread, spread 2 tablespoons of salsa. Spoon the chicken mixture evenly over the bread that has been covered with salsa. 1/4 cup Cheddar cheese should be on each sandwich.

Cook for 5 minutes, or until the cheese is melted and starting to color, under a preheated broiler.

GRILLED SHRIMP MARGARITA

4 servings | 15 minutes to prepare | 5 minutes to cook FACTS ABOUT THE NUTRITION

188 calories | 1.3 grams of carbohydrate | 11.1 grams of fat | 18.7 grams of protein | 173 milligrams of cholesterol

INGREDIENTS

2 teaspoons tequila 1 pound shrimp (peeled and deveined)

olive oil, 3 tablespoons

cayenne pepper, 1/4 teaspoon

3 tbsp cilantro, finely chopped

salt (quarter teaspoon)

lime juice, 2 tblsp.

4 bamboo skewers (20 minutes in water)

2 garlic cloves, chopped

DIRECTIONS

In a mixing bowl, combine the shrimp, olive oil, cilantro, lime juice, garlic, tequila, cayenne, and salt. Refrigerate the shrimp in the marinade for 30 minutes, covered with plastic wrap.

Preheat an outdoor grill to high heat and coat the grate lightly with oil.

Take the shrimp out of the bowl and thread them onto skewers; discard the marinade.

Cook for 2 to 3 minutes per side on a preheated grill until shrimp are pink.

Chapter Three

BASIL MAYO DRESSING FOR S ALAD

4 servings | 15 minutes to prepare | 10 minutes to cook

FACTS ABOUT THE NUTRITION

440 calories | 23.4 grams of carbs | 34.1 grams of fat | 12.2 grams of protein | 31 milligrams of cholesterol

INGREDIENTS

bacon (1 pound)

1/2 cup mayonnaise, 1 teaspoon salt

1 tsp pepper, ground

red wine vinegar, 2 tblsp

1 tbsp. oil from canola

1 tablespoon basil, finely chopped

1 pound of romaine lettuce, washed, dried, and torn into bite-size pieces

4 French bread slices, cut into 1/2-inch cubes

1 quart quartered cherry tomatoes

DIRECTIONS

In a big, deep skillet, brown the bacon. Cook until evenly browned on medium high heat. Drain, crumble, and set aside, with 2 tablespoons of the drippings set aside.

Whisk the reserved bacon drippings, mayonnaise, vinegar, and basil together in a small bowl and set aside at room temperature, covered.

Toss the bread with the salt and pepper in a large skillet set over medium heat. Drizzle with oil, tossing constantly, and cook until golden brown on medium-low heat.

Toss the romaine, tomatoes, bacon, and croutons together in a large mixing bowl. Toss the salad thoroughly with the dressing.

CORN SALAD IN THE SUMMER

4 servings | 25 minutes of prep time | 20 minutes of cooking time | 45 minutes total FACTS ABOUT THE NUTRITION

305 calories | 42.8 grams of carbs | 15.6 grams of fat | 6.2 grams of protein | 0 mg of cholesterol

INGREDIENTS

6 husked and cleaned ears of corn

olive oil, 1/4 cup

2 tablespoons white vinegar 3 large tomatoes (diced)

1 large onion, diced, seasoning to taste with salt and pepper

1 tablespoon basil, chopped

DIRECTIONS

Bring a large pot of water to a boil, lightly salted. Cook corn for 7 to 10 minutes in boiling water, or until tender. Drain and cool before using a sharp knife to cut the kernels from the cob.

Toss the corn, tomatoes, onions, basil, oil, vinegar, salt, and pepper together in a large mixing bowl. Place in the refrigerator until ready to use.

SANDWICHES OF ITALIAN GRILLED CHEESE

6 people | 8 minutes to prepare | 7 minutes to cook | 15 minutes total 394 calories | 42 grams of carbohydrates | 18.3 grams of fat | 15 grams of protein | 46 milligrams of cholesterol

INGREDIENTS

1 tbsp. butter (unsalted)

1 tsp. oregano (dried)

garlic powder, 1/8 teaspoon (optional)

1 package (8 ounces) shredded mozzarella

White bread, 12 slices

1 jar marinara sauce with vodka (24 oz)

DIRECTIONS

Turn on the broiler in your oven.

On a baking sheet, place 6 slices of bread. Each slice should be topped with a small handful of mozzarella cheese. The remaining 6 slices of bread will be used to finish the sandwich. Combine the butter and garlic powder in a small bowl, then brush or spread some over the tops of the sandwiches with the back of a spoon. Add oregano, if desired.

Broil for 2 to 3 minutes, or until golden brown, on a baking sheet. Remove the pan from the oven, flip the sandwiches, brush with butter, and sprinkle with oregano on the other side. Return to the broiler for another 2 minutes or until golden.

Serve immediately with a side of vodka sauce for dipping.

CHICKEN WRAPS THAT ARE SWEET AND SPICY

8 servings | 20 minutes to prepare | 15 minutes to cook

FACTS ABOUT THE NUTRITION

488 calories | 44.7 grams of carbs | 22.6 grams of fat | 26.6 grams of protein | 57 milligrams of cholesterol

INGREDIENTS

mayonnaise (half cup)

1 1/2 pound skinless, boneless chicken breast halves, thinly sliced

1 tablespoon seedless cucumber, finely chopped

1 cup salsa with a lot of chunks

honey, 1 tablespoon

honey, 1 tablespoon

cayenne pepper (1/2 teaspoon)

cayenne pepper (to taste) 1/2 teaspoon ground black pepper

flour tortillas, 8 (10 inch)

olive oil, 2 tablespoons

1 bag baby spinach leaves (10 ounces)

DIRECTIONS

In a bowl, combine the mayonnaise, cucumber, 1 tablespoon honey, 1/2 teaspoon cayenne pepper, and black pepper. Cover and chill until ready to use.

Cook and stir the chicken breast strips in the olive oil in a skillet over medium-high heat until golden and no longer pink in the middle, about 8 minutes. 1 tablespoon honey, 1/2 teaspoon cayenne pepper, and salsa Reduce the heat to low and continue to cook, stirring occasionally, for about 5 minutes, or until the flavors have blended.

Heat the tortillas in the microwave for 20 to 30 seconds per batch, 4 at a time, until warm and pliable.

Spread 1 tablespoon of the mayonnaise-cucumber mixture on each tortilla, then top with a layer of baby spinach leaves and 1/2 cup of the chicken mixture.

Begin rolling the burrito from the right side, folding the bottoms of each tortilla up about 2 inches. Fold the top of the tortilla down to enclose the filling and continue rolling to form a tight, compact cylinder when the burrito is half-rolled.

BRATS WITH BEER

10 servings | 5 minutes to prepare | 20 minutes to cook

FACTS ABOUT THE NUTRITION

382 calories | 9.7 grams of carbs | 27.4 grams of fat | 13.8 grams of protein | 69 milligrams of cholesterol

INGREDIENTS

4 beer cans (12 oz.)

garlic powder, 1 teaspoon

1 pound diced onion

1 tsp sodium

Bratwurst (bratwurst) (ten bratwurst

1 teaspoon black pepper, freshly ground

2 tsp. flakes de pimentón

DIRECTIONS

Preheat the grill to medium-high. Oil the grate when it's hot.

In a large pot, bring the beer and onions to a boil. Add the red pepper flakes, garlic powder, salt, and pepper to the bratwurst and submerge in the beer. Cook for an additional 10 to 12 minutes on medium heat. Remove the bratwurst from the beer mixture and continue to cook the onions on a low heat setting.

Cook the bratwurst for 5 to 10 minutes on a hot grill, turning once. As a topping or side dish, serve the beer mixture.

CARCASS SOUP WITH TTURKEY

12 servings | 45 minutes to prepare | 2 hours to cook
Calories: 133 | Carbohydrates: 27.7g | Fat: 1.3g | Protein: 4.2g | Cholesterol: 2mg NUTRITION FACTS Calories: 133 | Carbohydrates: 27.7g | Fat: 1.3g | Protein: 4.2g

INGREDIENTS

a carcass of turkey

Worcestershire sauce (1 tablespoon)

1 1/2 teaspoons salt 4 quarts water

6 tblsp. diced potatoes

1 tsp parsley, dry

4 oz. diced carrots

1 tsp basil powder

celery (diced) 2 stalks

1 onion, diced 1 bay leaf

1 tbsp. black pepper, freshly cracked

cabbage, shredded 1 1/2 cups

paprika (a quarter teaspoon)

1 whole peeled tomato can (28 ounces), chopped

1 tablespoon seasoning for poultry

1 cup barley, uncooked

1 tbsp thyme (dried)

DIRECTIONS

Place the turkey carcass in a large soup pot or stock pot and cover with water. Bring to a boil, then reduce to a low heat and cook the turkey frame for 1 hour, or until the remaining meat falls off the bones. Remove and chop any remaining turkey meat, as well as the turkey carcass. Meat should be chopped.

Fill a clean soup pot halfway with broth and strain through a fine mesh strainer. Stir in the potatoes, carrots, celery, onion, cabbage, tomatoes, barley, Worcestershire sauce, salt, parsley, basil, bay leaf, black pepper, paprika, poultry seasoning, and thyme to the strained broth. Bring to a boil, then reduce heat and add the potatoes, carrots, celery, onion, cabbage, tomatoes, barley, Worcestershire sauce, salt, parsley, basil, bay leaf, black pepper, paprika, poultry seasoning, and Continue to cook for another hour or until the vegetables are tender. Before serving, throw out the bay leaf.

SALMON SALAD WITH GREEK PASTA

8 servings | 20 minutes of prep time | 10 minutes of cooking time | 3 hours and 30 minutes total FACTS ABOUT THE NUTRITION

307 calories | 19.3 grams of carbs | 23.6 grams of fat | 5.4 grams of protein | 14 milligrams of cholesterol

INGREDIENTS

10 cherry tomatoes (halved) 2 cups penne pasta

red wine vinegar (quarter cup)

1 tablespoon lemon juice 1 small red onion (chopped)

2 teaspoons dried oregano 1 chopped green bell pepper 2 crushed garlic cloves 1 chopped red bell pepper

salt and pepper to taste, 1/2 cucumber, sliced

black olives, sliced 1/2 cup

2/3 cup olive oil (extra virgin)

feta cheese, crumbled

DIRECTIONS

Bring a large pot of lightly salted water to a boil over high heat. Bring the water back to a boil after adding the penne. Cook, uncovered, for about 11 minutes, or until the pasta is cooked through but still firm to the bite. Drain well in a colander in the sink after rinsing with cold water.

Vinegar, lemon juice, garlic, oregano, salt, pepper, and olive oil should all be whisked together. Remove the item from circulation.

In a large mixing bowl, toss together the pasta, tomatoes, onions, green and red peppers, cucumber, olives, and feta cheese. Toss the pasta in the vinaigrette and toss well. Before serving, cover with plastic wrap and chill for 3 hours.

CRANBERRY VINAIGRETTE IN A GREEN SALAD

8 people | 15 minutes to prepare | 5 minutes to cook | 20 minutes total 218 calories | 6.2 grams of carbohydrates | 19.2 grams of fat | 6.5 grams of protein | 11 milligrams of cholesterol

INGREDIENTS

2 tablespoons red wine vinegar 1 cup sliced almonds 1/2 teaspoon salt

1 teaspoon black pepper, freshly ground

olive oil, 1/3 cup

water, 2 tbsp

cranberries, fresh, 1/4 cup

thinly sliced red onion, 1/2

1 teaspoon mustard (Dijon)

4 oz. blue cheese (crumbled)

garlic, minced (1/2 teaspoon)

salad greens (1 pound)

DIRECTIONS

Preheat the oven to 375 degrees Fahrenheit (190 degrees Celsius) (190 degrees C). On a baking sheet, lay out almonds in a single layer. Preheat the oven to 350°F and toast the nuts for 5 minutes, or until they start to brown.

Add the vinegar, oil, cranberries, mustard, garlic, salt, pepper, and water to a blender or food processor and blend until smooth. Blend until the mixture is completely smooth.

Toss the almonds, onion, blue cheese, and greens with the vinegar mixture in a large mixing bowl until well combined.

STEAK SOUP | 8 SERVINGS | 45 MINUTES TO PREPARE | 1 HOUR 30 MINUTES TO COOK | 2 HOUR 15 MINUTES TO COOK

FACTS ABOUT THE NUTRITION

361 calories | 26.9 grams of carbs | 12.9 grams of fat | 36 grams of protein | 84 milligrams of cholesterol

4 chopped parsley sprigs

2 tbsp. oil

2 tbsp celery leaves (chopped)

1 1/2 pound boneless round steak, cubed

bay leaf (one)

1/2 c. onion, chopped

1 tsp. marjoram (dried)

all-purpose flour, 3 tblsp

1 1/2 cups diced, peeled carrots Potatoes, Yukon Gold

paprika, 1 tblsp.

12 CUP CARROTS, SLICED

1 tsp sodium

a half-cup of celery, chopped

black pepper, 1/4 teaspoon

1 tomato paste (6 oz.) can

1 (15.25 ounce) can whole kernel corn, drained 4 cups beef broth 1 (15.25 ounce) can beef broth

2 c.

DIRECTIONS

In a large skillet, melt butter and oil over medium heat until foam subsides, then add the steak cubes and onion. Cook, stirring occasionally, for about 10 minutes, or until the meat and onion have browned. Combine flour, paprika, salt, and pepper in a mixing bowl while the beef is cooking. Stir to coat the browned meat with the flour mixture.

Stir in the parsley, celery leaves, bay leaf, and marjoram to the beef broth and water in a large soup pot. Bring to a boil, stirring in the beef mixture. Reduce the heat to medium-low, cover the pot, and cook for 45 minutes, stirring occasionally.

Return the soup to a low heat and add the potatoes, carrots, celery, tomato paste, and corn; cook, uncovered, for 15 to 20 minutes, or until the vegetables are tender and the soup is thick. Serve immediately after removing the bay leaf.

SKILLET WITH CHICKEN, ASPARAGUS, AND MUSSELS

2 servings | 15 minutes of prep time | 25 minutes of cooking time | 40 minutes total 430 calories | 7.3 grams of carbohydrates | 33.5 grams of fat | 26.9 grams of protein | 107 milligrams of cholesterol

2 tbsp olive oil 1 1/2 tbsp lemon juice 1/4 teaspoon salt

1 1/2 tsp white cooking wine 1/2 teaspoon dried parsley

1 tsp basil powder

2 chicken breast halves (skinless, boneless) sliced

1 tsp oregano (dried)

trimmed and cut into thirds 1/2 pound fresh asparagus

garlic cloves, minced 1 1/2

1 c. fresh mushrooms, thinly sliced

DIRECTIONS

In a skillet over medium-high heat, melt the butter with the olive oil, then add the parsley, basil, oregano, garlic, salt, lemon juice, and wine. Cook and stir the chicken for about 3 minutes, or until it is browned. Reduce heat to medium-low and cook, stirring occasionally, for another 10 minutes, or until the chicken is no longer pink inside.

Add the asparagus and cook, stirring occasionally, for 3 minutes, or until bright green and just beginning to become tender. Cook for an additional 3 minutes, stirring frequently to allow the mushrooms to release their juices. Warm it up and serve.

Chapter Four

CAULIFLOWER SOUP WITH ROASTING

6 servings | 10 minutes of prep time | 1 hour of cooking time | 1 hour and 10 minutes of total time FACTS ABOUT THE NUTRITION

135 calories | 13.2 grams of carbs | 7.6 grams of fat | 4.4 grams of protein | 10 milligrams of cholesterol

INGREDIENTS

1 cauliflower head, florets cut

14 cup butter

2 tbsp extra-virgin olive oil with a roasted garlic flavor

1 chopped onion

1 tsp. nutmeg, ground

all-purpose flour, 3 tblsp

garlic powder, 2 teaspoons

1 chicken broth (14 oz.) can

salt (1 1/2 teaspoon)

1 quart of cream

1 teaspoon black pepper, freshly ground

1 tbsp. sherry (dried)

DIRECTIONS

Preheat the oven to 450 degrees Fahrenheit (230 degrees Celsius) (230 degrees C).

In a small roasting pan, put the cauliflower. Toss to coat with oil and nutmeg, garlic powder, salt, and pepper.

30 to 40 minutes in a preheated oven, roast the cauliflower, stirring every ten minutes, until golden brown and tender. Remove the dish from the oven and place it on a plate to cool.

In a large skillet over medium heat, melt the butter. Cook, stirring constantly, for about 10 minutes, until the onion is lightly golden brown.

Toss the onions in the flour to coat them. Pour the chicken broth and milk into the pan one cup at a time into the pan. Using a wire whisk, combine the flour and water until completely dissolved. Bring to a boil, stirring constantly, until the sauce thickens, then reduce to a low heat setting. Add the roasted cauliflower and sherry to the mix. Serve immediately, or blend half of the soup and recombine with the rest for a thicker consistency.

CHILI FOR DOGS THAT'S HOTTTTTTTTTTTTTTTTT

6 servings | 10 minutes of prep time | 20 minutes of cooking time | 30 minutes total FACTS ABOUT THE NUTRITION

168 calories | 7.5 grams of carbs | 9.4 grams of fat | 13.6 grams of protein | 47 milligrams of cholesterol

INGREDIENTS

ground beef, 1 pound

1/3 cup water 1/2 teaspoon black pepper 1/2 teaspoon salt

tomato sauce, half a can (10 oz.)

white sugar, 1/2 teaspoon

ketchup (half a cup)

1 teaspoon powdered onion

chili powder (2.5 teaspoons)

1 tsp. Worcestershire sauce (optional)

1. Place the ground beef in a large saucepan with enough water to cover it and mash it with a potato masher to break it up. Combine the tomato sauce, ketchup, chili powder, salt, black pepper, sugar, onion powder, and Worcestershire sauce in a large mixing bowl. Bring to a boil, then reduce to a low heat and cook for 20 minutes, or until the chili has slightly thickened and the beef is fully cooked.

SALAD WITH MANDARIN CHICKEN

6 people | 45 minutes to prepare | 8 minutes to cook | 53 minutes total FACTS ABOUT THE NUTRITION

425 calories | 44.7 grams of carbs | 18.9 grams of fat | 21.8 grams of protein | 35 milligrams of cholesterol

INGREDIENTS

1 tsp fresh ginger, finely chopped and peeled

1/2 cucumber sliced, scored, halved lengthwise, seeded

rice vinegar (about 1/3 cup)

red bell pepper, diced 1/2 cup

orange juice (about 1/3 cup)

1 tablespoon red onion, coarsely chopped

Vegetable oil, 1/4 cup

2 tomatoes, diced Roma

1 tsp. sesame oil (toasted)

shredded carrots 1

1 package dry onion soup mix (1 oz.)

1 fresh spinach (6 ounce) bag

2 tsp sugar, white

1 mandarin orange segment can (11 ounces), drained

1 garlic clove, squeezed

2 c. cooked chicken, diced

1 bow tie (farfalle) pasta package (8 ounces)

1 pound toasted sliced almonds

DIRECTIONS

To make the dressing, combine the ginger root, rice vinegar, orange juice, vegetable oil, sesame oil, soup mix, sugar, and garlic in a large mixing bowl and whisk until well combined. Cover and chill until ready to use.

Bring a large pot of water to a boil, lightly salted. Cook for 8 to 10 minutes, or until al dente, adding the bowtie pasta last. Drain and rinse under cold water. In a big mixing bowl, toss the pasta.

Toss the cucumbers, bell peppers, onions, tomatoes, carrots, spinach, mandarin oranges, chicken, and almonds with the pasta to make the salad. Toss the salad mixture with the dressing once more to evenly coat it. Right away, serve.

BANANA SANDWICH WITH GRILLED PEANUT BUTTER

1 serving | 2 minutes to prepare | 10 minutes to prepare | 12 minutes to cook 437 calories | 56.8 grams of carbohydrates | 18.7 grams of fat | 16.8 grams of protein | 0 milligrams of cholesterol

INGREDIENTS

sprayed on cooking
2 whole wheat sandwich slices
peanut butter, 2 tablespoons
a sliced banana

1. Spray a skillet or griddle with cooking spray and heat it over medium heat. On one side of each slice of bread, spread 1 tablespoon peanut butter. Place banana slices on one slice's peanut-butter side, top with the other slice, and firmly press together. 2 minutes per side, fry the sandwich until golden brown on both sides.

CHEESE SANDWICH WITH PESTO

1 serving | 5 minutes to prepare | 10 minutes to prepare | 15 minutes to cook FACTS ABOUT THE NUTRITION

503 calories | 24.2 grams of carbs | 36.5 grams of fat | 20.4 grams of protein | 82 milligrams of cholesterol

INGREDIENTS

Italian bread, 2 slices
Provolone cheese, 1 slice

2 tomato slices, divided 1 tablespoon softened butter

1 slice American cheese 1 tablespoon prepared pesto sauce

DIRECTIONS

Butter one side of a slice of bread and place it in a nonstick skillet over medium heat, buttered side down.

Place a slice of provolone cheese, tomato slices, and an American cheese slice on top of half of the pesto sauce in the skillet.

Place the second slice of bread, pesto side down, onto the sandwich and spread the remaining pesto sauce on one side. The top of the sandwich should be butter-coated.

5 minutes per side, gently fry the sandwich, flipping once, until both sides are golden brown and the cheese has melted.

SALAD WITH CHICKEN CLUB

6 servings | 20 minutes to prepare | 10 minutes to cook

FACTS ABOUT THE NUTRITION

485 calories | 37.1 grams of carbs | 30.1 grams of fat | 19.2 grams of protein | 48 milligrams of cholesterol

INGREDIENTS

pasta in the shape of a corkscrew, 8 oz.

Muenster cheese, cubed

1 cup salad dressing (Italian style)

1 celery pound

mayonnaise (quarter cup)

1 green bell pepper, chopped

8 ounces cherry tomatoes, halved 12 slices crispy cooked bacon, crumbled 2 cups chopped, cooked rotisserie chicken

1 peeled, pitted, and diced avocado

DIRECTIONS

Bring a large pot of water to a boil, lightly salted. Cook pasta in the boiling water, stirring occasionally until cooked through but firm to the bite, 10 to 12 minutes. Drain and rinse under cold water.

Whisk Italian-style dressing and mayonnaise together in a large bowl. Stir pasta, chicken, bacon, Muenster cheese, celery, green bell pepper, cherry tomatoes, and avocado into dressing until evenly coated.

BAKED MAC AND CHEESE FOR ONE

Servings: 1 | Prep: 10m | Cooks: 20m | Total: 30m NUTRITION FACTS

Calories: 496 | Carbohydrates: 30g | Fat: 30g | Protein: 19.8g | Cholesterol: 89mg

INGREDIENTS

3 tablespoons uncooked macaroni pasta

1/3 cup shredded Cheddar cheese

1 tablespoon butter

1/8 teaspoon ground mustard

1 tablespoon all-purpose flour

1 dash Worcestershire sauce

1/4 teaspoon salt

1 dash hot sauce

1 pinch pepper

1 teaspoon bread crumbs

1/8 teaspoon onion powder

1 tablespoon shredded Cheddar cheese

1/2 cup milk

DIRECTIONS

Preheat oven to 400 degrees Fahrenheit (200 degrees Celsius) (200 degrees C). 1 cup baking dish or oven-safe soup crock

Bring water to a boil in a small saucepan. Cook for approximately 8 minutes, stirring occasionally, until the macaroni is cooked but still firm to the biting. Drain well and save the water in a separate container.

Melt the butter in a medium-high-heat pot in the same way. Whisk together the flour, salt, pepper, onion powder, and milk until well combined. Cook for 2 minutes with stirring. Reduce to a low heat and add 1/3 cup cheese, mustard, Worcestershire sauce, and spicy sauce, whisking constantly. Add the macaroni that has been cooked. Fill the prepared dish halfway with macaroni and cheese. 1 tablespoon cheddar cheese, bread crumbs

Bake for 10 minutes, uncovered, until the cheese has melted and the macaroni is hot.

SOUP WITH RED LENTILS IN THE LEBANESE MANNER

8 servings | 20 minutes of prep time | 30 minutes of cooking time | 50 minutes total FACTS ABOUT THE NUTRITION

276 calories | 39.1 grams of carbs | 7 grams of fat | 16.7 grams of protein | 1 milligram of cholesterol

INGREDIENTS

6 cup stock (chicken)

1 pound red lentils, 1 tablespoon cumin powder

cayenne pepper (1/2 teaspoon)

olive oil, 3 tablespoons

1 pound cilantro, chopped

garlic, minced 1 tablespoon

lemon juice, 3/4 cup

1 sliced large onion

DIRECTIONS

In a large saucepan over high heat, bring chicken stock and lentils to a boil, then lower to medium-low heat, cover, and cook for 20 minutes.

In a skillet over medium heat, heat the olive oil. Stir in the garlic and onion, and cook for approximately 3 minutes, or until the onion is cooked and transparent.

Season with cumin and cayenne pepper and stir into the lentils. Simmer for another 10 minutes, or until lentils are cooked.

In a standing mixer or with a stick blender, carefully purée the soup until it is completely smooth. Before serving, toss in the cilantro and the lemon juice.

SALAD WITH FRESH CUCUMBER

8 servings | 10 minutes to prepare | 3 hours to cook | 3 hours and 10 minutes total FACTS ABOUT THE NUTRITION

320 calories | 6.9 grams of carbs | 32.9 grams of fat | 1.1 grams of protein | 16 milligrams of cholesterol

INGREDIENTS

2 peeled and thinly sliced big cucumbers

white sugar, 1 tablespoon

1 sliced sweet onion

1 tsp. dill weed (dried)

a pinch of salt

garlic powder, 1 teaspoon

1 teaspoon ground black pepper 1 1/2 cups mayonnaise, or more to taste

vinegar, 2 tbsp

DIRECTIONS

In a large mixing basin, combine cucumbers, sweet onion, and salt. Allow 30 minutes after covering dish with plastic wrap.

Place the cucumber mixture in a colander over a bowl or in the sink and drain for another 30 minutes, stirring periodically. Fill a large mixing bowl halfway with the drained cucumber mixture.

In a mixing bowl, whisk together the mayonnaise, vinegar, sugar, dill, garlic powder, and black pepper until smooth; pour over the cucumber mixture and toss to coat.

Refrigerate for at least 2 hours, covered in plastic wrap.

Servings: 4 | Prep: 20 minutes | Cooks: 20 minutes | Total: 40 minutes CHAKCHOUKA (SHAKSHOUKA) FACTS ABOUT THE NUTRITION

209 calories | 12.9 grams of carbs | 15 grams of fat | 7.8 grams of protein | 164 milligrams of cholesterol

INGREDIENTS

olive oil, 3 tablespoons

1 tsp cumin 1 tsp paprika 1 tsp paprika 1 tsp cumin 1 tsp cumin

1 cup bell peppers (any color) thinly sliced

1 tsp sodium

2 garlic cloves, minced

1 seeded and coarsely chopped spicy chile pepper, or as desired

2 1/2 c. tomatoes, chopped

A total of four eggs

DIRECTIONS

In a pan on medium heat, heat the olive oil. Cook, stirring occasionally, until the onion, bell peppers, and garlic have softened and the onion has gone translucent, approximately 5 minutes.

In a mixing basin, toss together the tomatoes, cumin, paprika, salt, and chilli pepper. Stir in the tomato mixture in the skillet.

Cook, covered, for approximately 10 minutes, or until the tomato juices have evaporated. In the tomato mixture, make four egg indentations. Into the indentations, crack the eggs. Allow the eggs to simmer for approximately 5 minutes, covered, until firm but not dry.

SOUP WITH SPICES AND SWEET POTATOES AND COCONUT

6 servings | 10 minutes to prepare | 55 minutes to cook 306 calories | 30.6 grams of carbohydrates | 20 grams of fat | 4.1 grams of protein | 0 milligrams of cholesterol

INGREDIENTS

1/2 pound sweet potatoes with orange flesh

1 tablespoon vegetable oil 3 cup vegetable broth

lemon juice (3.5 tblsp.)

a chopped onion

a pinch of salt

2 inch piece finely sliced fresh ginger root

1 tbsp. sesame oil (toasted)

red curry paste, 1 tbsp

1 tablespoon cilantro, chopped

1 unsweetened coconut milk can (15 oz.)

DIRECTIONS

Preheat the oven to 400 degrees Fahrenheit (200 degrees Celsius) (200 degrees C). Bake until the sweet potatoes are soft when pierced with a fork, approximately 45 minutes. Allow to cool after removing from oven.

Over medium heat, heat the oil in a large saucepan or soup pot. Cook and stir for 5 minutes, or until the onion and ginger are soft. Heat for 1 minute after stirring in the curry paste, then add the coconut milk and vegetable broth. Bring to a boil, then lower to a low heat and continue to cook for 5 minutes.

Cut the sweet potatoes into bite-sized slices after removing the skins. Add to the soup and simmer for a further 5 minutes to allow the flavors to meld. Season with salt after mixing in the lemon juice. Pour into bowls and top with sesame oil and cilantro.

SHRIMP AND GRITS is a dish that combines the flavors of shrimp and gri

4 servings | 25 minutes to prepare | 30 minutes to cook

FACTS ABOUT THE NUTRITION

434 calories | 33.2 grams of carbs | 19.5 grams of fat | 30.1 grams of protein | 226 milligrams of cholesterol

INGREDIENTS

4 bacon slices, quartered

peeled and deveined shrimp, 1 pound

water, 1/4 cup

a quarter teaspoon of Cajun seasoning

2 tbsp thick cream

12 tsp salt (or salt to taste)

lemon juice (2 teaspoons)

14 tsp black pepper, freshly ground

1 tsp. Worcestershire sauce (optional)

cayenne pepper, a sprinkle

water (four cups)

1 tsp. jalapeo pepper, minced

2 tbsp.

2 tbsp. green onion (minced)

1 tsp sodium

3 garlic cloves (chopped)

white grits, 1 cup

1 tsp fresh parsley, chopped

white Cheddar cheese, shredded

DIRECTIONS

Cook, stirring regularly, until nearly crisp, 5 to 7 minutes in a large pan over medium-high heat. Remove the bacon from the skillet and set it aside, leaving the drippings in the pan.

In a large mixing bowl, combine 1/4 cup water, cream, lemon juice, and Worcestershire sauce.

In a large saucepan, combine 4 cups water, 1 teaspoon salt, and bring to a boil. Stir grits into saucepan, come to a simmer, then lower to low heat and cook for 20 to 25 minutes, or until grits are creamy. Take the grits off the stove and mix in the white Cheddar cheese.

Season the shrimp with Cajun spice, 1/2 teaspoon salt, black pepper, and a dash of cayenne pepper in a large mixing bowl.

Over high heat, heat a skillet with the bacon drippings. In a single layer, cook shrimp for 1 minute in hot bacon grease. Cook for approximately 30 seconds after turning the shrimp and adding the jalapeño. Cook and stir until shrimp are cooked through, 3 to 4 minutes, adding water as needed to thin the sauce. Take the pan off the heat and add the parsley.

Toss the grits with the shrimp and sauce in a bowl.

STROMBOLIS QUICK AND EASY

3 servings | 10 minutes of prep time | 30 minutes of cooking time | 40 minutes total FACTS ABOUT THE NUTRITION

1065 calories | 77.8 grams of carbs | 54.6 grams of fat | 59 grams of protein | 162 milligrams of cholesterol

INGREDIENTS

pork sausage, 1/2 pound in bulk (optional)

American cheese, 4 slices

1 frozen loaf (1 pound) thawed bread dough

1 c. mozzarella cheese (shredded)

4 slices firm salami, to taste with salt and black pepper

1 egg white (lightly beaten) 4 slices thinly cut ham

DIRECTIONS

Preheat the oven to 425 degrees Fahrenheit (200 degrees Celsius) (220 degrees C).

Cook and stir sausage until it is crumbled, uniformly browned, and no longer pink in a large pan over medium-high heat, approximately 10 minutes. Any leftover grease should be drained and discarded.

On an oiled baking sheet, roll out the bread dough to a thickness of 3/4-inch. In the middle of the dough, lay pieces of salami, ham, and American cheese. Mozzarella cheese, salt, and pepper, as well as cooked sausage, should be sprinkled on top. Wrap the dough over the contents, squeezing and closing the corners to avoid leaking; brush with egg white on top.

Bake in a preheated oven for 17 to 20 minutes, or until the dough is gently browned.

ORZO BASIL WITH SUN-DRIED TOMATO

8 servings | 15 minutes to prepare | 8 minutes to cook Calories: 255 | Carbohydrates: 38.8g | Fat: 6.9g | Protein: 10g | Cholesterol: 7mg NUTRITION FACTS Calories: 255 | Carbohydrates: 38.8g | Fat: 6.9g | Protein: 10g

INGREDIENTS

3/4 cup grated Parmesan cheese 1/2 cup chopped fresh basil leaves 2 cups uncooked orzo pasta

salt, 1/2 teaspoon

1/3 cup sunflower seeds, chopped

-tomatillos seca

1 teaspoon black pepper, freshly ground

olive oil, 2 tablespoons

DIRECTIONS

Bring a big saucepan of water to a boil, lightly salted. Cook for 8 to 10 minutes, or until orzo is al dente, adding water as needed. Set aside after draining.

In a food processor, combine the basil and sun-dried tomatoes. 4 or 5 pulses until well combined.

Toss orzo, basil-tomato combination, olive oil, Parmesan cheese, salt, and pepper together in a large mixing dish. Warm or cold options are available.

SQUASH SOUP WITH SPICED BUTTERNUTS

8 servings | 45 minutes to prepare | 20 minutes to cook | 1 hour and 15 minutes total FACTS ABOUT THE NUTRITION

298 calories | 45.2 grams of carbs | 10.6 grams of fat | 7.1 grams of protein | 34 milligrams of cholesterol

INGREDIENTS

3 pounds halved and seeded butternut squash

1/8 tsp allspice powder

2 tbsp.

1/8 tsp. nutmeg, powdered

1 sliced medium onion

8 tsp ginger powder

salt and pepper to taste 1 leek, sliced

2 garlic cloves (slice)

sherry wine, half a cup

2 chicken broth cans (49.5 fluid ounces)

1 cup cream (half-n-half)

peeled and quartered 2 big russet potatoes

sour cream, 1/2 cup (optional)

cayenne pepper (1/8 teaspoon)

DIRECTIONS

Preheat the oven to 375°F/190°C/190°C/190°C/190°C (190 degrees C). A baking dish or a cookie sheet with sides should have a thin coating of water in it. Cut side down on the platter, place the squash halves. Preheat the oven to 400°F and bake for 40 minutes, or until a fork easily pierces the flesh. Remove the peel when it has cooled a little. Remove the item from circulation.

In a big saucepan over medium heat, melt the butter. Cook for a few minutes, or until the onion, leek, and garlic are soft. In a large saucepan, add the chicken broth. Bring to a boil with the potatoes. Cook for 20 minutes, or until the potatoes are tender. Mash the squash and potatoes together until the pieces are tiny. Puree the soup in stages in a blender or food processor, or use an immersion hand blender to puree the soup. Toss the pot back in.

Stir in the sherry and half-and-half cream after seasoning with cayenne pepper, allspice, nutmeg, ginger, salt, and pepper. Bring to a boil, but don't overheat. Top with a spoonful of sour cream and serve in bowls.

WINGS WITH HONEY AND GARLIC FROM KRISTA

8 servings | 10 minutes of prep time | 50 minutes of cooking time | 1 hour total 337 calories | 35.1 grams of carbohydrate | 13.4 grams of fat | 19.1 grams of protein | 58 milligrams of cholesterol

INGREDIENTS

split and discarded tips off 24 chicken wings

honey, 5 tbsp

3/4 cup brown sugar, tightly packed

1 tablespoon soy sauce (low sodium)

minced garlic cloves (5 cloves)

cornstarch, 3 tblsp

1 tsp ginger root, chopped

water, 3/4 cup

2 1/2 quarts liquid

BACON, MUSHROOMS, AND ONIONS IN A SOUTHERN FRIED CABBAGE

10 servings | 15 minutes to prepare | 30 minutes to cook

FACTS ABOUT THE NUTRITION

123 calories | 9.6 grams of carbs | 6.4 grams of fat | 8 grams of protein | 16 milligrams of cholesterol

INGREDIENTS

bacon (one pound)

8 oz. fresh mushrooms, sliced

1 big head of cabbage, salt & pepper to taste

1 sliced large onion

DIRECTIONS

Cook, turning periodically, until uniformly browned, approximately 10 minutes, in a large pan over medium-high heat. Using paper towels, drain the bacon pieces and crumble when cold. Remove all of the bacon drippings from the pan except 3 tablespoons.

In the leftover bacon drippings, cook and toss the cabbage, onion, and mushrooms until they are soft and lightly browned, approximately 20 minutes. In a large mixing bowl, combine the cabbage, bacon, and salt and pepper to taste Salt & pepper to taste.

SWISS SANDWICHES WITH TANGY TURKEY

4 servings | 15 minutes to prepare | 10 minutes to cook 856 calories | 42.6 grams of carbohydrate | 58.9 grams of fat | 41.9 grams of protein | 154 milligrams of cholesterol

INGREDIENTS

1 red onion, chopped

6 tbsp. softened butter

1 tbsp. thyme (dried)

roast turkey, 1 pound, thinly sliced

mayonnaise (half cup)

Tomato, 8 slices

brown mustard, coarse-grain

Swiss cheese, 8 slices

8 slices of French bread in a rural style

DIRECTIONS

Mix the red onion, thyme, mayonnaise, and mustard together in a small mixing basin. On one side of each piece of bread, spread a little amount of this mixture. Using the other side of the bread pieces, spread butter on the other side.

Over medium heat, warm a large skillet. 4 pieces of bread, butter side down, in a pan 1/4 of the sliced turkey, 2 slices of tomato, and 2 slices of Swiss cheese should be layered on each piece of bread. Place the butter-side up on the remaining pieces of bread. Flip the sandwiches over when the bottoms are golden brown. Cook until the second side is golden brown.

WRAPS OF BLT

4 servings | 15 minutes to prepare | 10 minutes to cook
FACTS ABOUT THE NUTRITION

695 calories | 64.2 grams of carbs | 34.1 grams of fat | 31.4 grams of protein | 71 milligrams of cholesterol

INGREDIENTS

1 pound thickly sliced bacon, 1 inch cubes

4 (12-inch) flour tortillas 1/2 head iceberg lettuce, shredded a diced tomato

1 cup grated cheese Cheddar cheese is a type of cheese that originated in the United

DIRECTIONS

In a big, deep skillet, brown the bacon. Cook until evenly browned on medium-high heat. Set aside after draining.

On a microwave-safe plate, place one tortilla. 1/4 cup cheese, strewn across tortilla Cook for 1 to 2 minutes in the microwave, or until the cheese has melted. Add 1/4 of the bacon, lettuce, and tomato to the top of the sandwich right away. Fold the tortilla's sides inwards and roll it up. With the remaining ingredients, repeat the process. Before serving, cut the wraps in half.

CHIMICANGAS WITH BEEF

6 people | 15 minutes to prepare | 25 minutes to cook | 40 minutes total FACTS ABOUT THE NUTRITION

369 calories | 15.8 grams of carbs | 25.4 grams of fat | 19.7 grams of protein | 70 milligrams of cholesterol

INGREDIENTS

ground beef, 1 pound

1 can green chilies, chopped (4 oz.)

1 finely chopped small onion

2 tbsp. white vinegar, distilled

1 garlic clove (chopped)

1 cup grated cheese Cheddar cheese is a type of cheese that originated in the United

1/2 teaspoon taco seasoning mix, or more according to personal preference

margarine, 1/4 cup

1 tsp. oregano (dried)

6 corn tortillas (each 7 inches wide)

sour cream, 1/4 cup

DIRECTIONS

Preheat the oven to 450 degrees Fahrenheit (230 degrees Celsius) (230 degrees C).

In a skillet over medium heat, brown the ground beef, onion, garlic, taco seasoning, and oregano, about 8 minutes, breaking the meat up into crumbles. Excess fat is removed. Combine the sour cream, chilies, and vinegar in a large mixing bowl. Remove the pan from the heat and stir in the Cheddar.

In a small skillet on low heat, melt the margarine. Dip each tortilla for about 30 seconds in the melted margarine, or until soft. Fill the tortilla with about 1/3 cup of the meat mixture and place it on a baking sheet. Fold the right and left sides of the tortilla over the filling, then the top and bottom, enclosing the filling completely. On the baking sheet, place the tortilla, seam side down. Fill the tortillas with the remaining filling and repeat the process.

Preheat the oven to 350°F and bake the tortilla for 15 minutes, or until crisp.

RICE SOUP WITH WILD TURKEY

8 servings | 20 minutes to prepare | 1 hour to cook | 1 hour and 20 minutes total FACTS ABOUT THE NUTRITION

252 calories | 14.4 grams of carbs | 15.2 grams of fat | 14.3 grams of protein | 61 milligrams of cholesterol

INGREDIENTS

1/3 cup shredded carrot 2/3 cup wild rice, uncooked

2 c.

2 c. turkey, chopped

butter, 6 tbsp

salt to taste (1/2 teaspoon kosher salt)

1 tablespoon onion, finely chopped

1/2 teaspoon black pepper powder (or to taste)

a quarter-cup of celery, finely chopped

slivered almonds, 1/4 cup

a third of a cup of flour (all-purpose)

lemon juice (1/2 teaspoon)

3/4 cup half-and-half cream 4 cups turkey stock

DIRECTIONS

In a saucepan, bring water and wild rice to a boil. Reduce to a low heat, cover, and cook for 40 to 45 minutes, or until the rice is tender but not mushy. Drain any excess liquid, fluff the rice with a fork, and continue to cook for another 5 minutes, uncovered. Set aside the rice that has been cooked.

In a soup pot on medium heat, melt the butter. Cook for about 5 minutes, stirring occasionally, until the onion is translucent. Cook for 3 to 5 minutes, stirring constantly, until the flour is pale yellowish-brown in color. Whisk in the turkey stock in a slow, steady stream until there are no lumps of flour. Add the carrot and stir to combine. Bring the mixture to a low simmer, whisking constantly, for another 2 minutes, or until the stock is thick and smooth and the carrots are tender.

Add the wild rice, turkey, salt, pepper, and almonds to the mixture and mix well. Return to a low heat and cook for an additional 2 minutes to thoroughly heat the ingredients. Add the lemon juice and half bring the soup to a boil. Serve immediately.

SALAD WITH SPINACH AND BASIL.

10 servings | 15 minutes to prepare | 15 minutes to cook
FACTS ABOUT THE NUTRITION

372 calories | 36.4 grams of carbs | 20.7 grams of fat | 13.6 grams of protein | 15 milligrams of cholesterol

INGREDIENTS

4 oz. prosciutto, diced 1 (16 oz.) package bow tie pasta

1 spinach leaves (6 oz.) package

To taste, season with salt and black pepper.

2 c basil leaves, fresh

Parmesan cheese, freshly grated

1/2 cup olive oil (extra virgin)

half-cup pine nuts, toasted

3 garlic cloves (chopped)

DIRECTIONS

Bring a large pot of lightly salted water to a boil over high heat. Stir in the bow tie pasta and return to a boil once the water has reached a boil. Cook, uncovered, for about 12 minutes, or until the pasta is cooked through but still firm to the bite. To cool down, give it a good rinsing with cold water. Drain thoroughly in a sink colander.

In a large mixing bowl, combine the basil and spinach.

In a skillet over medium heat, heat the olive oil; cook and stir the garlic for 1 minute, then add the prosciutto and cook for another 2 to 3 minutes. Turn off the burner. Toss in the spinach and basil mixture in a large mixing bowl. Retoss the pasta after it has been drained. Using salt and pepper, season to taste. To serve, garnish with pine nuts and Parmesan cheese.

PINE NUTS, SAGE, AND ROMANO IN SPAGHETTI SQUASH

4 servings | 10 minutes to prepare | 50 minutes to cook

FACTS ABOUT THE NUTRITION

150 calories | 13.7 grams of carbs | 9.4 grams of fat | 5.6 grams of protein | 13 milligrams of cholesterol

INGREDIENTS

1 halved and seeded spaghetti squash

2 tbsp. fresh sage (chopped)

2 teaspoons butter, melted 1/4 cup toasted pine nuts

Salt and pepper to taste 1/4 cup grated Pecorino Romano cheese

DIRECTIONS

Preheat the oven to 350 degrees Fahrenheit (180 degrees Celsius) (175 degrees C).

In a large baking dish, place the squash, cut side down.

Cook the squash for 50 minutes in a preheated oven.

Using a fork, scrape the squash flesh from the rind into a bowl. Toss to combine the pine nuts, cheese, sage, butter, salt, and pepper. Right away, serve.

DOGS THAT HAVE BEEN RECENT

8 servings | 10 minutes of prep time | 15 minutes of cooking time | 25 minutes total FACTS ABOUT THE NUTRITION

313 calories | 13.2 grams of carbs | 23.8 grams of fat | 10.2 grams of protein | 37 milligrams of cholesterol

INGREDIENTS

Hot dogs for 8 people

1 refrigerated crescent dinner roll (8 oz.) from Pillsbury

4 American cheese slices, cut into 6 strips each

DIRECTIONS

Preheat the oven to 375°F. Using a sharp knife, slit the hot dogs to within 1/2 inch of the ends, then insert three strips of cheese into each slit.

Make triangles from the dough. Each hot dog is wrapped in a dough triangle. Place, cheese side up, on an ungreased cookie sheet.

Preheat the oven to 350°F and bake for 12 to 15 minutes, or until golden brown.

PUMPERNICKEL BREAD BREAD MACHINE

12 servings | 10 minutes of prep time | 3 hours and 45 minutes of cooking time | 3 hours and 55 minutes of total time

FACTS ABOUT THE NUTRITION

119 calories | 22.4 grams of carbohydrate | 2.3 grams of fat | 3.4 grams of protein | 0 milligrams of cholesterol

INGREDIENTS

1 and a quarter cup of hot water

1/2 cup flour for bread

1 1/2 tbsp. oil

rye flour (1 cup)

Molasses, 1/3 cup

1 cup flour made from whole grains

cocoa powder 3 tbsp

1 1/2 tsp. wheat gluten (optional)

caraway seeds, 1 tablespoon (optional)

2 1/2 tblsp yeast (for bread machine)

salt (1 1/2 teaspoon)

1. Place the ingredients in the bread machine pan in the manufacturer's recommended order. Press Start after selecting the Basic cycle.

PUMPKIN SOUP WITH COCONUT CURRY

6 servings | 20 minutes to prepare | 30 minutes to cook

FACTS ABOUT THE NUTRITION

171 calories | 12 grams of carbohydrate | 13.5 grams of fat | 2 grams of protein | 0 milligrams of cholesterol

INGREDIENTS

coconut oil (1/4 cup)

1 cup chopped onions 1 teaspoon salt

1 tsp coriander (ground)

1 garlic clove (chopped)

1 tsp red pepper flakes (crushed)

3 c. broth

1 pure pumpkin (15 oz.) can

curry powder, 1 teaspoon

1 coconut milk (light) cup

In a large pot over medium-high heat, heat the coconut oil. Cook until the onions are translucent, about 5 minutes, after adding the onions and garlic. Add the vegetable broth, curry powder, salt, coriander, and red pepper flakes, and stir to combine. Cook, stirring constantly, for about 10 minutes, until the mixture reaches a gentle boil. Cook for another 15 to 20 minutes, covered, with occasional stirring. Cook for 5 more minutes, whisking in the pumpkin and coconut milk.

Fill a blender halfway with soup and process until smooth, working in batches if needed. Before serving, return to a pot and reheat for a few minutes over medium heat.

SALAD WITH BRAISED CARROT

6 Servings | 20 minutes to prepare | 30 minutes to cook | 1 hour and 30 minutes total 295 calories | 23.8 grams of carbohydrates | 19.7 grams of fat | 7.6 grams of protein | 14 milligrams of cholesterol

INGREDIENTS

1 teaspoon honey 1/2 cup slivered almonds 2 pounds peeled and thinly sliced carrots on the diagonal

1 tsp. vinegar

2 garlic cloves, chopped

cranberries, dried, 1/3 cup

extra-virgin olive oil (about 1/4 cup)

1 (4 oz) package crumbled Danish blue cheese salt and pepper to taste

Arugula, 2 cups

DIRECTIONS

Preheat oven to 400 degrees Fahrenheit (200 degrees Celsius) (200 degrees C).

In a large mixing bowl, mix together the carrots, almonds, and garlic. Season to taste with salt and pepper after drizzling with olive oil. Place on a baking sheet that has not been greased.

30 minutes in a preheated oven, bake the carrots until soft and brown on the edges. Allow to cool to room temperature before removing from the oven.

Return the carrots to the mixing bowl once they have cooled, and drizzle with honey and vinegar, tossing to coat. Toss in the cranberries and blue cheese until thoroughly combined. Serve immediately with arugula.

SLOPPY JOES IN TONYA'S WORLD

4 servings | 10 minutes to prepare | 30 minutes to cook 362 calories | 31.2 grams of carbohydrates | 15.3 grams of fat | 23.7 grams of protein | 71 milligrams of cholesterol

INGREDIENTS

2 lb. beef mince

1 1/2 tsp. Worcestershire

1 teaspoon vinegar, 1/2 cup chopped onion

1 celery stalk, chopped

1 teaspoon powdered mustard

ketchup (7 oz.)

lemon juice (1/8 teaspoon)

brown sugar (1 tablespoon)

8 hamburger buns (white or wheat).

DIRECTIONS

Over medium-high heat, place a large skillet. In a large pan, crumble the ground meat; add the onion and celery. Cook, stirring constantly, for 7 to 10 minutes, or until the meat is thoroughly browned.

In a large mixing bowl, combine the meat, ketchup, brown sugar, Worcestershire sauce, vinegar, mustard, and lemon juice. Reduce heat to medium-low and continue to cook, stirring occasionally, until the sauce has thickened and the mixture is heated, approximately 20 minutes.

GRILLED CHEESE SANDWICH WITH A JALAPENO POPPER

2 servings | 10 minutes to prepare | 10 minutes to prepare | 10 minutes to cook | 20 minutes total 528 calories | 40.9 grams of carbohydrates | 34 grams of fat | 16.5 grams of protein | 89 milligrams of cholesterol

INGREDIENTS

softened 2 oz. cream cheese

butter, 4 tsp

sour cream, 1 tblsp

8 crumpled tortilla chips

10 jalapeño pepper slices, chopped, or to taste

1 pound shredded cheese Colby-Monterey Jack is a cheese made by combining the flavors of Colby and Monterey

Sandwich rolls made with ciabatta

DIRECTIONS

In a small mixing bowl, mix together the cream cheese, sour cream, and pickled jalapeo. Remove the item from circulation. Preheat the skillet to medium.

Each roll should be cut in half horizontally, then the rounded tops of the ciabatta rolls should be sliced off to produce a flat top half. 1 teaspoon butter on the doughy cut side of the bottom bun, 1 teaspoon butter on the now-flattened top bun On the unbuttered side of the bottom bun, spread half of the cream cheese mixture, half of the crumbled chips, and half of the shredded cheese. Place the sandwich on the heated pan and top with the remaining half of the bread. Make a second sandwich and repeat the process.

Grill until gently cooked on one side and golden brown on the other, 3 to 5 minutes.

SOUP WITH LEEK AND ROASTED CAULIFLOWER

6 servings | 10 minutes of prep time | 1 hour and 5 minutes of cooking time | 1 hour and 15 minutes total FACTS ABOUT THE NUTRITION

209 calories | 15.4 grams of carbohydrate | 15.9 grams of fat | 3.8 grams of protein | 34 milligrams of cholesterol

INGREDIENTS

2 garlic cloves, chopped

chicken stock (1 quart)

2 tbsp. oil

heavy whipping cream (about a third of a cup)

florets from 1 head of cauliflower

1 tsp chervil (dry)

butter, 3 tablespoons

1 tbsp. salt (kosher)

2 chopped leeks (just the white portion)

1 teaspoon black pepper, freshly cracked

1 tablespoon flour, all-purpose

DIRECTIONS

Preheat the oven to 375°F/190°C/190°C/190°C/190°C (190 degrees C).

In a small bowl, combine garlic and vegetable oil. Place the cauliflower florets on a baking pan and drizzle with the oil mixture. Toss to evenly distribute the ingredients.

30 minutes in a preheated oven, bake cauliflower until soft and gently browned.

Cook and whisk leeks and flour in melted butter in a 4-quart stockpot over medium heat until aromatic and thoroughly mixed, 5 to 10 minutes. Simmer for 20 to 25 minutes, until the cauliflower, chicken stock, and cream have mixed. Stir in the chervil, salt, and pepper, and continue to cook for 10 to 15 minutes longer, or until the soup reaches the desired thickness.

BACON AND BEANS

6 servings | 15 minutes of prep time | 2 hours and 20 minutes of cooking time | 2 hours and 35 minutes of total time FACTS ABOUT THE NUTRITION

631 calories | 52.2 grams of carbs | 35.3 grams of fat | 26.6 grams of protein | 51 milligrams of cholesterol

INGREDIENTS

1 bay leaf 9 cups water 1 (16 ounce) container dry navy beans

1 pound bacon 1 tablespoon salt

black pepper, 1/4 teaspoon

1/8 teaspoon ground garlic cloves 2 chopped onions

1 (16 oz.) container diced tomatoes 2 celery stalks, chopped

4 tsp bouillon de poulet de poulet de poulet de poulet de water (four cups)

DIRECTIONS

Boil the beans for an hour in 9 cups of water. Set aside after draining.

Cook the bacon until it reaches your preferred texture (soft or crisp, as desired), then drain all except 1/4 cup of the fat. The bacon should be coarsely chopped.

In the reserved bacon fat, sauté the onions and celery until tender, but do not drain. Simmer for 2 hours with the chicken stock or cubes, 4 cups water, beans, bay leaf, salt, pepper, and cloves.

Combine the tomatoes and their juice in a large mixing bowl. Serve.

SALAD DE POTATOES

20 servings | 20 minutes to prepare | 10 minutes to cook

FACTS ABOUT THE NUTRITION

339 calories | 20.4 grams of carbs | 27.6 grams of fat | 4.1 grams of protein | 53 milligrams of cholesterol

INGREDIENTS

5 lb. chopped red potatoes

1 celery stalk, chopped

mayonnaise (three cups)

3 tsp mustard (prepared)

2 c. pickled cucumbers, coarsely chopped

1 TBS ACV

1 teaspoon salt (or to taste) 5 hard-boiled eggs, diced

1 red onion, chopped

1 teaspoon black pepper, freshly ground

DIRECTIONS

Bring salted water to a boil over potatoes in a big saucepan. Reduce the heat to mediumlow and continue to cook for another 10 minutes, or until the vegetables are soft. Drain. While the dressing is being made, return the potatoes to the empty saucepan to dry. salt

In a large mixing bowl, combine the mayonnaise, pickles, hard-boiled eggs, red onion, celery, mustard, cider vinegar, 1 teaspoon salt, and pepper. In a large mixing bowl, combine the potatoes and mayonnaise. Before serving, refrigerate the dish for at least six hours or overnight.

SHRIMP OF CAJUN

4 servings | 5 minutes to prepare | 5 minutes to prepare | 5 minutes to cook | 10 minutes total FACTS ABOUT THE NUTRITION

166 calories | 0.9 grams of carbohydrate | 5 grams of fat | 28 grams of protein | 259 milligrams of cholesterol

INGREDIENTS

paprika, 1 tblsp.

black pepper, 1/4 teaspoon

dried thyme, 3/4 teaspoon

cayenne pepper, 1/4 teaspoon (or more to taste)

1 tsp. oregano (dried)

peeled and deveined 1 1/2 pounds big shrimp

garlic powder, 1/4 teaspoon

1 tsp. oil

salt (quarter teaspoon)

DIRECTIONS

In a sealable plastic bag, mix together the paprika, thyme, oregano, garlic powder, salt, pepper, and cayenne pepper. Shake to coat shrimp.

In a large nonstick skillet, heat the oil on medium high. Cook and stir shrimp in hot oil for approximately 4 minutes, or until they are brilliant pink on the exterior and the flesh is no longer translucent in the middle.

POTATO SOUP WITH MANDI'S CHEESE

5 people | 10 minutes to prepare | 35 minutes to cook | 45 minutes total FACTS ABOUT THE NUTRITION

466 calories | 51 grams of carbs | 21.5 grams of fat | 18.7 grams of protein | 45 milligrams of cholesterol

INGREDIENTS

3 tablespoons margarine, melted 5 peeled and diced potatoes

1 finely sliced carrot

all-purpose flour, 3 tblsp

finely sliced celery stalk

steak seasoning (1 1/2 teaspoons)

1 teaspoon black pepper 1 1/2 cup water

1 tsp sodium

2 cups four-cheese shredded mixture

milk, 2 1/2 c.

DIRECTIONS

Toss potatoes, carrots, celery, water, and salt in a large saucepan over medium heat. Bring to a boil, then lower to a low heat, cover, and cook for 15 to 20 minutes, until the potatoes are cooked. Stir in the milk when the vegetables are soft.

Melted margarine, flour, steak seasoning, and pepper should all be combined in a small basin. Stir into the soup, then boil, stirring constantly, until thick and bubbling. Remove the pan from the heat and toss in the cheese until it is completely melted. Before serving, set aside for 5 to 10 minutes.

FRIED RICE WITH THAI SPICY BASIL CHICKEN

6 servings | 30 minutes of prep time | 10 minutes of cooking time | 40 minutes total 794 calories | 116.4 grams of carbohydrates | 22.1 grams of fat | 29.1 grams of protein | 46 milligrams of cholesterol

INGREDIENTS

oyster sauce (3 tablespoons)

1 pound chicken breast, boneless and skinless, cut into thin strips

2 tsp. soy sauce

1 finely sliced and seeded red pepper

1 tsp. sugar

1 finely sliced onion (about 1 cup)

frying oil: 1/2 cup peanut

2 c Thai basil, sweet

4 cups cooked and cooled jasmine rice

1 slice of cucumber (optional)

garlic cloves, smashed, 6 big cloves

cilantro sprigs (half a cup) (optional)

crushed serrano peppers

DIRECTIONS

In a large mixing basin, combine the oyster sauce, fish sauce, and sugar.

In a wok, heat the oil until it starts to smoke over medium-high heat. Stir rapidly to incorporate the garlic and serrano peppers. Cook, stirring constantly, until the chicken is no longer pink, adding the bell pepper, onion, and oyster sauce combination. Raise the heat to high and immediately whisk in the cold rice, making sure the sauce is well combined. Break apart any rice that's stuck together using the back of a spoon.

Take the pan off the heat and add the basil leaves. As desired, garnish with cucumber slices and cilantro.

SMOKED SAUSAGE WITH CABBAGE PASTA

6 people | 15 minutes to prepare | 20 minutes to cook | 35 minutes total 845 calories | 68.5 grams of carbohydrate | 51.2 grams of fat | 30.9 grams of protein | 95 milligrams of cholesterol

INGREDIENTS

1 farfalle (bow tie) pasta (16 ounce package)

1 big shredded head of green cabbage

1 tablespoon of butter

to taste with salt and pepper

2 garlic cloves, chopped

1 pound thinly sliced smoked sausage

olive oil, 1/4 cup

Parmesan cheese (grated): 1/4 cup

DIRECTIONS

Bring a big saucepan of lightly salted water to a boil over high heat. Stir in the bow tie spaghetti and bring to a boil once the water has reached a boil. Cook, uncovered, for approximately 12 minutes, or until the pasta is cooked through but still firm to the biting. Drain well in a sink colander.

In a big saucepan over medium heat, melt the butter. Season with salt and pepper, then add the garlic, olive oil, and cabbage. Cook for 15 minutes, or until the cabbage is soft. Cook for another 5 minutes, or until the sausage and bow tie pasta are fully warm. Serve immediately, topped with Parmesan cheese.

BUTTERNUT SQUASH SOUP WITH CARAMELIZED BUTTERNUT

12 people | 20 minutes to prepare | 30 minutes to cook | 50 minutes total Calories: 189 | Carbohydrates: 24.9g | Fat: 10.3g | Protein: 2.9g | Cholesterol: 23mg NUTRITION FACTS Calories: 189 | Carbohydrates: 24.9g | Fat: 10.3g | Protein: 2.9g

INGREDIENTS

extra-virgin olive oil, 3 tblsp.

4 cup chicken broth (or more if necessary)

1/4 cup honey 3 pounds peeled and diced butternut squash

1 chopped big onion

heavy whipping cream (1/2 cup)

butter, 3 tablespoons

1 tsp. nutmeg powder, or to taste

1 tbsp. salt (to taste)

1 teaspoon white pepper, freshly cracked, to taste

DIRECTIONS

In a big saucepan over high heat, heat olive oil. In a heated skillet, cook and stir squash for approximately 10 minutes, or until it is thoroughly browned. Cook and toss the squash with the onion, butter, sea salt, and cracked white pepper for approximately 10 minutes, or until the onions are totally soft and starting to brown.

Bring the chicken stock and honey to a boil over the squash, then lower to a low heat and cook for 5 minutes, or until the squash is soft.

Fill a blender just halfway with the mixture. Cover and secure the lid, then pulse a few times to combine. Until smooth, puree in batches.

To serve, whisk together the cream, nutmeg, salt, and freshly ground white pepper.

TOMATO SOUP WITH ROASTED INGREDIENTS

NUTRITION FACTS: 6 SERVINGS | 10 MINUTES TO PREPARE | 50 MINUTES TO COOK

140 calories | 14.7 grams of carbs | 7.6 grams of fat | 5.4 grams of protein | 3 milligrams of cholesterol

INGREDIENTS

1 1/2 teaspoon freshly ground black pepper 3 pounds roma (plum) tomatoes, quartered

1 half-and-quartered yellow onion

3 garlic cloves, quartered

5 cups chicken broth (low sodium) 1/2 red bell pepper, diced olive oil, 3 tablespoons

2 tsp. basil powder

a pinch of salt

1 tsp parsley, dry

DIRECTIONS

Preheat the oven to 400 degrees Fahrenheit (200 degrees Celsius) (200 degrees C). Wrap aluminum foil around a large baking sheet.

On the prepared baking sheet, arrange the tomatoes, onion, and red bell pepper in one layer. Season with salt and pepper and drizzle olive oil over tomato mixture.

Cook for 30 minutes in a preheated oven; add the garlic and roast for another 15 minutes, or until the tomato mixture is soft.

In a large stockpot, bring the chicken broth, basil, and parsley to a boil; decrease heat to low and continue to cook.

In a blender, puree half of the tomato sauce. Cover and let aside; pulse a few times before blending until smooth, adding a tiny amount of heated chicken broth if necessary. Fill a stockpot halfway with chicken broth and purée the tomato mixture. Half of the tomato combination should be pureed and added to the chicken stock mixture. 5 minutes on low heat

MELT IN THE CALIFORNIA

4 servings | 15 minutes to prepare | 2 minutes to cook FACTS ABOUT THE NUTRITION

335 calories | 21.1 grams of carbs | 22.5 grams of fat | 15.6 grams of protein | 26 milligrams of cholesterol

INGREDIENTS

4 pieces gently toasted wholegrain bread

toasted almonds, 1/3 cup

1 cup sliced mushrooms 1 avocado (sliced) 1 tomato (sliced)

Swiss cheese, 4 pieces

DIRECTIONS

Preheat the broiler on high in the oven.

On a baking pan, place the toasted bread. 1/4 avocado, mushrooms, almonds, and tomato slices are spread on each piece of bread. A piece of Swiss cheese should be placed on top of each.

Broil the open-face sandwiches for approximately 2 minutes, or until the cheese starts to melt and bubble. Warm sandwiches should be served.

VERY EASY AND QUICK DUMPLINGS WITH CHICKEN

6 people | 5 minutes to prepare | 15 minutes to cook | 20 minutes total FACTS ABOUT THE NUTRITION

361 calories | 29.6 grams of carbs | 15.1 grams of fat | 25 grams of protein | 63 milligrams of cholesterol

INGREDIENTS

2 14 cup baking powder

2/3 cup milk 2 cans (14 ounce) chicken broth

2 drained chunk chicken cans (10 ounces)

DIRECTIONS

Combine the biscuit mix and milk in a medium mixing dish and whisk until combined. Remove the item from circulation.

Bring the chicken broth and the cans of chicken broth to a boil in a saucepan together. Take a handful of biscuit dough and flatten it in your hands after the broth has reached a steady boil. Cut 1 to 2 inch pieces and place them into the simmering soup. At the very least, make sure they are completely submerged. When all of the dough has been added to the saucepan, gently stir to ensure that the broth covers the newest dough clumps. Cover and cook, stirring periodically, for 10 minutes over medium heat.

BURGERS WITH VEGAN BLACK BEAN

4 servings | 15 minutes to prepare | 20 minutes to prepare | 35 minutes total FACTS ABOUT THE NUTRITION

264 calories | 51.7 grams of carbs | 1.4 grams of fat | 11.6 grams of protein | 0 milligrams of cholesterol

INGREDIENTS

1 can (15 ounces) drained and rinsed black beans

1 tsp cayenne

1 cup sweet onion, chopped

cumin powder (1 teaspoon)

garlic, minced 1 tablespoon

1 tsp. sea salt (such as Old Bay)

3 peeled and shredded baby carrots (optional)

salt (quarter teaspoon)

green bell pepper, minced 1/4 cup (optional)

black pepper, 1/4 teaspoon

cornstarch (1 tablespoon)

2 slices whole-wheat bread, shredded

1 tsp. water

a third of a cup of unbleached flour, or more if required

3 tablespoons chile-garlic sauce (Sriracha, for example), or to taste

DIRECTIONS

Preheat the oven to 350 degrees Fahrenheit (180 degrees Celsius) (175 degrees C). Preheat the oven to 350°F. Prepare a baking sheet by greasing it.

In a mixing basin, combine the black beans, onion, garlic, carrots, and green bell pepper; mash well. Mix.

In a separate small mixing bowl, combine cornstarch, water, chile-garlic sauce, chili powder, cumin, seafood seasoning, salt, and black pepper. In a separate bowl, whisk together the cornstarch and water. Add the cornstarch mixture to the black bean mixture and

Combine the beans with the whole-wheat bread. 1/4 cup flour at a time, until a sticky batter develops, stir flour into bean mixture.

Using a 3/4-inch thickness per mound, spoon burger-sized mounds of batter onto the prepared baking sheet. To make burgers, combine all of the ingredients in a bowl and form into

Cook for approximately 10 minutes on each side in a preheated oven until the center is done and the exterior is crisp.

SOUP WITH ASPARAGUS CREAM AND MUSSELS

8 people | 15 minutes to prepare | 40 minutes to cook | 55 minutes total FACTS ABOUT THE NUTRITION

171 calories | 12.7 grams of carbs | 11.8 grams of fat | 5.2 grams of protein | 29 milligrams of cholesterol

INGREDIENTS

3 bacon slivers

1 tablespoon bacon drippings (6 cups chicken broth)

peeled and diced 1 potato

1 teaspoon of butter

1 pound asparagus spears, tips and stalks set aside chopped

3 celery stalks, salt and pepper to taste

1 chopped onion

8 oz. fresh mushrooms, sliced

all-purpose flour, 3 tblsp

a third of a cup of half-and-half

DIRECTIONS

Cook, turning occasionally, until evenly browned, about 10 minutes, in a large, deep skillet over medium-high heat. On a paper towel–lined plate, drain the bacon slices. When the bacon is cool enough to handle, crumble it and place it aside. 1 tablespoon bacon drippings should be kept aside.

In a saucepan over medium heat, melt butter and drippings.

In a large saucepan, cook and stir celery and onion for 4 minutes, or until onion is translucent.

Cook for 1 minute while whisking in the flour.

Bring to a boil, whisking in chicken broth.

Reserving the asparagus tips for later, add the potato and chopped asparagus stalks. Salt and black pepper to taste.

Simmer for 20 minutes after lowering the heat.

Fill a blender halfway with soup. Using a folded kitchen towel to hold down the lid of the blender, carefully start it, using a few quick pulses to get the soup moving before leaving it on to puree. In a clean pot, puree in batches until smooth. You can also puree the soup in the cooking pot with a stick blender.

In the same skillet as the bacon, cook and stir mushrooms and asparagus tips until liquid has evaporated, about 5 to 8 minutes. If necessary, season with salt and pepper.

To make the pureed soup, add the mushrooms, asparagus tips, and half-and-half cream. Cook until everything is completely warm.

Crumbled bacon can be used to garnish the soup.

SLOW-COOKER CHILI WITH VEGAN INGREDIENTS

15 servings | 45 minutes of preparation time | 5 hours and 10 minutes of cooking time | 5 hours and 55 minutes of total time Calories: 134 | Carbohydrates: 24.8g | Fat: 2.4g | Protein: 6.3g | Cholesterol: 0mg NUTRITION FACTS Calories: 134 | Carbohydrates: 24.8g | Fat: 2.4g | Protein: 6.3g

INGREDIENTS

1 teaspoon of extra virgin olive oil

1 tbsp. oregano (dried)

1 finely chopped green bell pepper

1 tsp parsley powder

1/2 teaspoon salt, 1 red bell pepper, chopped

1/2 teaspoon ground black pepper 1 yellow bell pepper (chopped)

2 chopped onions 2 diced tomatoes with juice (14.5 oz.)

1 (15 oz) can black beans, rinsed and drained 4 garlic cloves, minced

1 cup frozen corn kernels, thawed 1 (15 ounce) can kidney beans, rinsed and drained 1 (10 ounce) package frozen chopped spinach, thawed and drained

2 (6 oz.) cans tomato paste 1 zucchini, chopped

1 (8-ounce) can tomato sauce (or more if needed) 1 yellow squash, chopped

chili powder, 6 tbsp

1 cup vegetable broth, plus a little extra if necessary

cumin powder (1 tablespoon)

DIRECTIONS

Cook the green, red, and yellow bell peppers, onions, and garlic in olive oil in a large skillet over medium heat for 8 to 10 minutes, or until the onions begin to brown. In a slow cooker, place the mixture. Toss in the spinach, corn, zucchini, yellow squash, chili powder, cumin, oregano, parsley, salt, black pepper, tomatoes, black beans, garbanzo beans, kidney beans, and tomato paste until everything is well combined. Toss the ingredients with the tomato sauce and vegetable broth.

Cook on low for 4 to 5 hours, or until all of the vegetables are tender. Check for seasoning; if the chili is too thick, add more tomato sauce and vegetable broth until it reaches the desired consistency. To blend the flavors, cook for an additional 1 to 2 hours.

SALAD WITH QUINOA AND VEGANS

12 servings | 20 minutes of prep time | 25 minutes of cooking time | 1 hour and 30 minutes of total time FACTS ABOUT THE NUTRITION

148 calories | 22.9 grams of carbohydrate | 4.5 grams of fat | 4.6 grams of protein | 0 milligrams of cholesterol

INGREDIENTS

1 tsp. oil from canola

half a cucumber, diced

garlic, minced 1 tablespoon

thawed corn kernels, 1/2 cup

a quarter cup chopped (yellow or purple) onion

red onion, diced

1 1/2 tablespoons fresh chopped cilantro 2 1/2 cups water

1 tablespoon chopped fresh mint 2 teaspoons salt (or to taste)

black pepper, 1/4 teaspoon

1 tsp sodium

quinoa, 2 cup

black pepper, 1/4 teaspoon

fresh tomato, diced

olive oil, 2 tablespoons

carrots, 3/4 cup diced

balsamic vinegar, 3 tablespoons

yellow bell pepper, diced

DIRECTIONS

In a saucepan on medium heat, heat the canola oil. 5 minutes in the hot oil, cook and stir the garlic and 1/4 cup onion until the onion softens and turns translucent. Bring the water, 2 teaspoons salt, and 1/4 teaspoon black pepper to a boil, then add the quinoa and cover. Cook for about 20 minutes, or until quinoa is tender. Transfer the quinoa to a large mixing bowl after draining any remaining water with a mesh strainer. Allow to cool before serving.

In a chilled quinoa bowl, mix together the tomato, carrots, bell pepper, cucumber, corn, and 1/4 cup red onion. 1 teaspoon salt, 1/4 teaspoon black pepper, cilantro, mint, 1 teaspoon salt Pour the olive oil and balsamic vinegar over the salad and toss gently to combine.

RESTAURANT-STYLE ITALIAN SUBSCRIPTIONS

8 servings | 20 minutes to prepare | 1 hour to cook | 1 hour and 20 minutes total FACTS ABOUT THE NUTRITION

708 calories | 40.4 grams of carbs | 47.3 grams of fat | 29.2 grams of protein | 79 milligrams of cholesterol

INGREDIENTS

1 rinsed and torn head red leaf lettuce

red pepper flakes (1/4 teaspoon)

2 c. chopped fresh tomatoes

1 tsp oregano (dried)

1 finely chopped medium red onion

Capacola sausage, sliced, 1/2 pound

olive oil (six tablespoons)

Genoa salami, 1/2 pound thinly sliced

white wine vinegar, 2 tblsp

2 tablespoons fresh parsley, chopped 1/4 pound thinly sliced prosciutto

Provolone cheese, sliced, 1/2 pound

4 submarine rolls, split 2 garlic cloves (chopped)

1 tsp basil powder

1 cup slices of dill pickle

DIRECTIONS

Combine the lettuce, tomatoes, and onion in a large mixing bowl. Combine the olive oil, white wine vinegar, parsley, garlic, basil, red pepper flakes, and oregano in a separate bowl and whisk to combine. Toss the salad to evenly coat it with the dressing. 1 hour in the refrigerator

Layer the Capacola, salami, prosciutto, and provolone cheese evenly on each submarine roll. Add some salad and as many pickle slices as you'd like. Close and serve the rolls.

JIM'S ONION SODA WITH CHEDDAR BREAD

12 people | 15 minutes to prepare | 30 minutes to cook | 55 minutes total FACTS ABOUT THE NUTRITION

264 calories | 36.9 grams of carbs | 9.1 grams of fat | 8.2 grams of protein | 24 milligrams of cholesterol

INGREDIENTS

1 1/4 cup buttermilk 4 cups bread flour + more for dusting

2 tbsp. confectioners' sugar 1 1/2 tsp. salt

1 tbsp flour

onion, finely chopped (approximately 3/4 cup)

6 tbsp. softened butter

Cheddar cheese, shredded

DIRECTIONS

Preheat the oven to 425 degrees Fahrenheit (200 degrees Celsius) (220 degrees C). Use parchment paper to cover a baking sheet.

Combine bread flour, salt, and baking powder in a large mixing bowl and whisk until well combined. To make a dough, combine the butter, buttermilk, and confectioners' sugar; add the onion and Cheddar cheese and gently combine. Make two balls out of the dough by dividing it in half. Flatten the loaves to about 2 inches thick on the prepared baking sheet. Make a flour dusting on each loaf.

Preheat the oven to 350°F and bake for 30 minutes, or until golden brown. Cool for a few minutes on wire racks before serving.

Chapter Five

SOUP WITH SPICES AND SWEET POTATOES AND COCONUT

6 servings | 10 minutes to prepare | 55 minutes to cook 306 calories | 30.6 grams of carbohydrates | 20 grams of fat | 4.1 grams of protein | 0 milligrams of cholesterol

INGREDIENTS

1/2 pound sweet potatoes with orange flesh

1 tablespoon vegetable oil 3 cup vegetable broth

lemon juice (3.5 tblsp.)

a chopped onion

a pinch of salt

2 inch piece finely sliced fresh ginger root

1 tbsp. sesame oil (toasted)

red curry paste, 1 tbsp

1 tablespoon cilantro, chopped

1 unsweetened coconut milk can (15 oz.)

DIRECTIONS

SOUP WITH SPICES AND SWEET POTATOES AND COCONUT

Preheat the oven to 400 degrees Fahrenheit (200 degrees Celsius) (200 degrees C). Bake until the sweet potatoes are soft when pierced with a fork, approximately 45 minutes. Allow to cool after removing from oven.

Over medium heat, heat the oil in a large saucepan or soup pot. Cook and stir for 5 minutes, or until the onion and ginger are soft. Heat for 1 minute after stirring in the curry paste, then add the coconut milk and vegetable broth. Bring to a boil, then lower to a low heat and continue to cook for 5 minutes.

Cut the sweet potatoes into bite-sized slices after removing the skins. Add to the soup and simmer for a further 5 minutes to allow the flavors to meld. Season with salt after mixing in the lemon juice. Pour into bowls and top with sesame oil and cilantro.

SHRIMP AND GRITS is a dish that combines the flavors of shrimp and gri

4 servings | 25 minutes to prepare | 30 minutes to cook

FACTS ABOUT THE NUTRITION

434 calories | 33.2 grams of carbs | 19.5 grams of fat | 30.1 grams of protein | 226 milligrams of cholesterol

INGREDIENTS

4 bacon slices, quartered

peeled and deveined shrimp, 1 pound

water, 1/4 cup

a quarter teaspoon of Cajun seasoning

2 tbsp thick cream

12 tsp salt (or salt to taste)

lemon juice (2 teaspoons)

14 tsp black pepper, freshly ground

1 tsp. Worcestershire sauce (optional)

cayenne pepper, a sprinkle

water (four cups)

1 tsp. jalapeo pepper, minced

2 tbsp.

2 tbsp. green onion (minced)

1 tsp sodium

3 garlic cloves (chopped)

white grits, 1 cup

1 tsp fresh parsley, chopped

white Cheddar cheese, shredded

DIRECTIONS

Cook, stirring regularly, until nearly crisp, 5 to 7 minutes in a large pan over medium-high heat. Remove the bacon from the skillet and set it aside, leaving the drippings in the pan.

In a large mixing bowl, combine 1/4 cup water, cream, lemon juice, and Worcestershire sauce.

In a large saucepan, combine 4 cups water, 1 teaspoon salt, and bring to a boil. Stir grits into saucepan, come to a simmer, then lower to low heat and cook for 20 to 25 minutes, or until grits are creamy. Take the grits off the stove and mix in the white Cheddar cheese.

Season the shrimp with Cajun spice, 1/2 teaspoon salt, black pepper, and a dash of cayenne pepper in a large mixing bowl.

Over high heat, heat a skillet with the bacon drippings. In a single layer, cook shrimp for 1 minute in hot bacon grease. Cook for approximately 30 seconds after turning the shrimp and adding the jalapeño. Cook and stir until shrimp are cooked through, 3 to 4 minutes, adding water as needed to thin the sauce. Take the pan off the heat and add the parsley.

Toss the grits with the shrimp and sauce in a bowl.

STROMBOLIS QUICK AND EASY

3 servings | 10 minutes of prep time | 30 minutes of cooking time | 40 minutes total FACTS ABOUT THE NUTRITION

1065 calories | 77.8 grams of carbs | 54.6 grams of fat | 59 grams of protein | 162 milligrams of cholesterol

INGREDIENTS

pork sausage, 1/2 pound in bulk (optional)

American cheese, 4 slices

1 frozen loaf (1 pound) thawed bread dough

1 c. mozzarella cheese (shredded)

4 slices firm salami, to taste with salt and black pepper

1 egg white (lightly beaten) 4 slices thinly cut ham

DIRECTIONS

Preheat the oven to 425 degrees Fahrenheit (200 degrees Celsius) (220 degrees C).

Cook and stir sausage until it is crumbled, uniformly browned, and no longer pink in a large pan over medium-high heat, approximately 10 minutes. Any leftover grease should be drained and discarded.

On an oiled baking sheet, roll out the bread dough to a thickness of 3/4-inch. In the middle of the dough, lay pieces of salami, ham, and American cheese. Mozzarella cheese, salt, and pepper, as well as cooked sausage, should be sprinkled on top. Wrap the dough over the contents, squeezing and closing the corners to avoid leaking; brush with egg white on top.

Bake in a preheated oven for 17 to 20 minutes, or until the dough is gently browned.

ORZO BASIL WITH SUN-DRIED TOMATO

8 servings | 15 minutes to prepare | 8 minutes to cook
Calories: 255 | Carbohydrates: 38.8g | Fat: 6.9g | Protein: 10g | Cholesterol: 7mg NUTRITION FACTS Calories: 255 | Carbohydrates: 38.8g | Fat: 6.9g | Protein: 10g

INGREDIENTS

3/4 cup grated Parmesan cheese 1/2 cup chopped fresh basil leaves 2 cups uncooked orzo pasta

salt, 1/2 teaspoon

1/3 cup sunflower seeds, chopped

-tomatillos seca

1 teaspoon black pepper, freshly ground

olive oil, 2 tablespoons

DIRECTIONS

Bring a big saucepan of water to a boil, lightly salted. Cook for 8 to 10 minutes, or until orzo is al dente, adding water as needed. Set aside after draining.

In a food processor, combine the basil and sun-dried tomatoes. 4 or 5 pulses until well combined.

Toss orzo, basil-tomato combination, olive oil, Parmesan cheese, salt, and pepper together in a large mixing dish. Warm or cold options are available.

SQUASH SOUP WITH SPICED BUTTERNUTS

8 servings | 45 minutes to prepare | 20 minutes to cook | 1 hour and 15 minutes total FACTS ABOUT THE NUTRITION

298 calories | 45.2 grams of carbs | 10.6 grams of fat | 7.1 grams of protein | 34 milligrams of cholesterol

INGREDIENTS

3 pounds halved and seeded butternut squash

1/8 tsp allspice powder

2 tbsp.

1/8 tsp. nutmeg, powdered

1 sliced medium onion

8 tsp ginger powder

salt and pepper to taste 1 leek, sliced

2 garlic cloves (slice)

sherry wine, half a cup

2 chicken broth cans (49.5 fluid ounces)

1 cup cream (half-n-half)

peeled and quartered 2 big russet potatoes

sour cream, 1/2 cup (optional)

cayenne pepper (1/8 teaspoon)

DIRECTIONS

Preheat the oven to 375°F/190°C/190°C/190°C/190°C (190 degrees C). A baking dish or a cookie sheet with sides should have a thin coating of water in it. Cut side down on the platter, place the squash halves. Preheat the oven to 400°F and bake for 40 minutes, or until a fork easily pierces the flesh. Remove the peel when it has cooled a little. Remove the item from circulation.

In a big saucepan over medium heat, melt the butter. Cook for a few minutes, or until the onion, leek, and garlic are soft. In a large saucepan, add the chicken broth. Bring to a boil with the potatoes. Cook for 20 minutes, or until the potatoes are tender. Mash the squash and potatoes together until the pieces are tiny. Puree the soup in stages in a blender or food processor, or use an immersion hand blender to puree the soup. Toss the pot back in.

Stir in the sherry and half-and-half cream after seasoning with cayenne pepper, allspice, nutmeg, ginger, salt, and pepper. Bring to a boil, but don't overheat. Top with a spoonful of sour cream and serve in bowls.

WINGS WITH HONEY AND GARLIC FROM KRISTA

8 servings | 10 minutes of prep time | 50 minutes of cooking time | 1 hour total 337 calories | 35.1 grams of carbohydrate

SOUP WITH SPICES AND SWEET POTATOES AND COCONUT

| 13.4 grams of fat | 19.1 grams of protein | 58 milligrams of cholesterol

INGREDIENTS

split and discarded tips off 24 chicken wings

honey, 5 tbsp

3/4 cup brown sugar, tightly packed

1 tablespoon soy sauce (low sodium)

minced garlic cloves (5 cloves)

cornstarch, 3 tblsp

1 tsp ginger root, chopped

water, 3/4 cup

2 1/2 quarts liquid

BACON, MUSHROOMS, AND ONIONS IN A SOUTHERN FRIED CABBAGE

10 servings | 15 minutes to prepare | 30 minutes to cook

FACTS ABOUT THE NUTRITION

123 calories | 9.6 grams of carbs | 6.4 grams of fat | 8 grams of protein | 16 milligrams of cholesterol

INGREDIENTS

bacon (one pound)

8 oz. fresh mushrooms, sliced

1 big head of cabbage, salt & pepper to taste

1 sliced large onion

DIRECTIONS

Cook, turning periodically, until uniformly browned, approximately 10 minutes, in a large pan over medium-high heat. Using paper towels, drain the bacon pieces and crumble when cold. Remove all of the bacon drippings from the pan except 3 tablespoons.

In the leftover bacon drippings, cook and toss the cabbage, onion, and mushrooms until they are soft and lightly browned, approximately 20 minutes. In a large mixing bowl, combine the cabbage, bacon, and salt and pepper to taste Salt & pepper to taste.

SWISS SANDWICHES WITH TANGY TURKEY

4 servings | 15 minutes to prepare | 10 minutes to cook 856 calories | 42.6 grams of carbohydrate | 58.9 grams of fat | 41.9 grams of protein | 154 milligrams of cholesterol

INGREDIENTS

1 red onion, chopped

6 tbsp. softened butter

1 tbsp. thyme (dried)

roast turkey, 1 pound, thinly sliced

mayonnaise (half cup)

Tomato, 8 slices

brown mustard, coarse-grain

Swiss cheese, 8 slices

8 slices of French bread in a rural style

DIRECTIONS

Mix the red onion, thyme, mayonnaise, and mustard together in a small mixing basin. On one side of each piece of bread, spread a little amount of this mixture. Using the other side of the bread pieces, spread butter on the other side.

Over medium heat, warm a large skillet. 4 pieces of bread, butter side down, in a pan 1/4 of the sliced turkey, 2 slices of tomato, and 2 slices of Swiss cheese should be layered on each piece of bread. Place the butter-side up on the remaining pieces of bread. Flip the sandwiches over when the bottoms are golden brown. Cook until the second side is golden brown.

WRAPS OF BLT

4 servings | 15 minutes to prepare | 10 minutes to cook

FACTS ABOUT THE NUTRITION

695 calories | 64.2 grams of carbs | 34.1 grams of fat | 31.4 grams of protein | 71 milligrams of cholesterol

INGREDIENTS

1 pound thickly sliced bacon, 1 inch cubes

4 (12-inch) flour tortillas 1/2 head iceberg lettuce, shredded

a diced tomato

1 cup grated cheese Cheddar cheese is a type of cheese that originated in the United

DIRECTIONS

In a big, deep skillet, brown the bacon. Cook until evenly browned on medium-high heat. Set aside after draining.

On a microwave-safe plate, place one tortilla. 1/4 cup cheese, strewn across tortilla Cook for 1 to 2 minutes in the microwave, or until the cheese has melted. Add 1/4 of the bacon, lettuce, and tomato to the top of the sandwich right away. Fold the tortilla's sides inwards and roll it up. With the remaining ingredients, repeat the process. Before serving, cut the wraps in half.

CHIMICANGAS WITH BEEF

6 people | 15 minutes to prepare | 25 minutes to cook | 40 minutes total FACTS ABOUT THE NUTRITION

369 calories | 15.8 grams of carbs | 25.4 grams of fat | 19.7 grams of protein | 70 milligrams of cholesterol

INGREDIENTS

ground beef, 1 pound

1 can green chilies, chopped (4 oz.)

1 finely chopped small onion

2 tbsp. white vinegar, distilled

1 garlic clove (chopped)

1 cup grated cheese Cheddar cheese is a type of cheese that originated in the United

1/2 teaspoon taco seasoning mix, or more according to personal preference

margarine, 1/4 cup

1 tsp. oregano (dried)

6 corn tortillas (each 7 inches wide)

sour cream, 1/4 cup

DIRECTIONS

Preheat the oven to 450 degrees Fahrenheit (230 degrees Celsius) (230 degrees C).

SOUP WITH SPICES AND SWEET POTATOES AND COCONUT

In a skillet over medium heat, brown the ground beef, onion, garlic, taco seasoning, and oregano, about 8 minutes, breaking the meat up into crumbles. Excess fat is removed. Combine the sour cream, chilies, and vinegar in a large mixing bowl. Remove the pan from the heat and stir in the Cheddar.

In a small skillet on low heat, melt the margarine. Dip each tortilla for about 30 seconds in the melted margarine, or until soft. Fill the tortilla with about 1/3 cup of the meat mixture and place it on a baking sheet. Fold the right and left sides of the tortilla over the filling, then the top and bottom, enclosing the filling completely. On the baking sheet, place the tortilla, seam side down. Fill the tortillas with the remaining filling and repeat the process.

Preheat the oven to 350°F and bake the tortilla for 15 minutes, or until crisp.

RICE SOUP WITH WILD TURKEY

8 servings | 20 minutes to prepare | 1 hour to cook | 1 hour and 20 minutes total FACTS ABOUT THE NUTRITION

252 calories | 14.4 grams of carbs | 15.2 grams of fat | 14.3 grams of protein | 61 milligrams of cholesterol

INGREDIENTS

1/3 cup shredded carrot 2/3 cup wild rice, uncooked

2 c.

2 c. turkey, chopped

butter, 6 tbsp

salt to taste (1/2 teaspoon kosher salt)

1 tablespoon onion, finely chopped

1/2 teaspoon black pepper powder (or to taste)

a quarter-cup of celery, finely chopped

slivered almonds, 1/4 cup

a third of a cup of flour (all-purpose)

lemon juice (1/2 teaspoon)

3/4 cup half-and-half cream 4 cups turkey stock

DIRECTIONS

In a saucepan, bring water and wild rice to a boil. Reduce to a low heat, cover, and cook for 40 to 45 minutes, or until the rice is tender but not mushy. Drain any excess liquid, fluff the rice with a fork, and continue to cook for another 5 minutes, uncovered. Set aside the rice that has been cooked.

In a soup pot on medium heat, melt the butter. Cook for about 5 minutes, stirring occasionally, until the onion is translucent. Cook for 3 to 5 minutes, stirring constantly, until the flour is pale yellowish-brown in color. Whisk in the turkey stock in a slow, steady stream until there are no lumps of flour. Add the carrot and stir to combine. Bring the mixture to a low simmer, whisking constantly, for another 2 minutes, or until the stock is thick and smooth and the carrots are tender.

Add the wild rice, turkey, salt, pepper, and almonds to the mixture and mix well. Return to a low heat and cook for an additional 2 minutes to thoroughly heat the ingredients. Add the lemon juice and half bring the soup to a boil. Serve immediately.

SALAD WITH SPINACH AND BASIL.

10 servings | 15 minutes to prepare | 15 minutes to cook

FACTS ABOUT THE NUTRITION

372 calories | 36.4 grams of carbs | 20.7 grams of fat | 13.6 grams of protein | 15 milligrams of cholesterol

INGREDIENTS

4 oz. prosciutto, diced 1 (16 oz.) package bow tie pasta

1 spinach leaves (6 oz.) package

To taste, season with salt and black pepper.

2 c basil leaves, fresh

Parmesan cheese, freshly grated

1/2 cup olive oil (extra virgin)

half-cup pine nuts, toasted

3 garlic cloves (chopped)

DIRECTIONS

Bring a large pot of lightly salted water to a boil over high heat. Stir in the bow tie pasta and return to a boil once the water has reached a boil. Cook, uncovered, for about 12 minutes, or until the pasta is cooked through but still firm to the bite. To cool down, give it a good rinsing with cold water. Drain thoroughly in a sink colander.

In a large mixing bowl, combine the basil and spinach.

In a skillet over medium heat, heat the olive oil; cook and stir the garlic for 1 minute, then add the prosciutto and cook for another 2 to 3 minutes. Turn off the burner. Toss in the spinach and basil mixture in a large mixing bowl. Retoss the pasta after it has been drained. Using salt and pepper, season to taste. To serve, garnish with pine nuts and Parmesan cheese.

PINE NUTS, SAGE, AND ROMANO IN SPAGHETTI SQUASH

4 servings | 10 minutes to prepare | 50 minutes to cook

FACTS ABOUT THE NUTRITION

150 calories | 13.7 grams of carbs | 9.4 grams of fat | 5.6 grams of protein | 13 milligrams of cholesterol

INGREDIENTS

1 halved and seeded spaghetti squash

2 tbsp. fresh sage (chopped)

2 teaspoons butter, melted 1/4 cup toasted pine nuts

Salt and pepper to taste 1/4 cup grated Pecorino Romano cheese

DIRECTIONS

Preheat the oven to 350 degrees Fahrenheit (180 degrees Celsius) (175 degrees C).

In a large baking dish, place the squash, cut side down.

Cook the squash for 50 minutes in a preheated oven.

Using a fork, scrape the squash flesh from the rind into a bowl. Toss to combine the pine nuts, cheese, sage, butter, salt, and pepper. Right away, serve.

DOGS THAT HAVE BEEN RECENT

8 servings | 10 minutes of prep time | 15 minutes of cooking time | 25 minutes total FACTS ABOUT THE NUTRITION

313 calories | 13.2 grams of carbs | 23.8 grams of fat | 10.2 grams of protein | 37 milligrams of cholesterol

INGREDIENTS

Hot dogs for 8 people

1 refrigerated crescent dinner roll (8 oz.) from Pillsbury

4 American cheese slices, cut into 6 strips each

DIRECTIONS

Preheat the oven to 375°F. Using a sharp knife, slit the hot dogs to within 1/2 inch of the ends, then insert three strips of cheese into each slit.

Make triangles from the dough. Each hot dog is wrapped in a dough triangle. Place, cheese side up, on an ungreased cookie sheet.

Preheat the oven to 350°F and bake for 12 to 15 minutes, or until golden brown.

PUMPERNICKEL BREAD BREAD MACHINE

12 servings | 10 minutes of prep time | 3 hours and 45 minutes of cooking time | 3 hours and 55 minutes of total time

FACTS ABOUT THE NUTRITION

119 calories | 22.4 grams of carbohydrate | 2.3 grams of fat | 3.4 grams of protein | 0 milligrams of cholesterol

INGREDIENTS

1 and a quarter cup of hot water

1/2 cup flour for bread

1 1/2 tbsp. oil

rye flour (1 cup)

Molasses, 1/3 cup

1 cup flour made from whole grains

cocoa powder 3 tbsp

1 1/2 tsp. wheat gluten (optional)

caraway seeds, 1 tablespoon (optional)

2 1/2 tblsp yeast (for bread machine)

salt (1 1/2 teaspoon)

1. Place the ingredients in the bread machine pan in the manufacturer's recommended order. Press Start after selecting the Basic cycle.

PUMPKIN SOUP WITH COCONUT CURRY

6 servings | 20 minutes to prepare | 30 minutes to cook

FACTS ABOUT THE NUTRITION

171 calories | 12 grams of carbohydrate | 13.5 grams of fat | 2 grams of protein | 0 milligrams of cholesterol

INGREDIENTS

coconut oil (1/4 cup)

1 cup chopped onions 1 teaspoon salt

1 tsp coriander (ground)

1 garlic clove (chopped)

1 tsp red pepper flakes (crushed)

3 c. broth

1 pure pumpkin (15 oz.) can

curry powder, 1 teaspoon

1 coconut milk (light) cup

In a large pot over medium-high heat, heat the coconut oil. Cook until the onions are translucent, about 5 minutes, after adding the onions and garlic. Add the vegetable broth, curry powder, salt, coriander, and red pepper flakes, and stir to combine. Cook, stirring constantly, for about 10 minutes, until the mixture reaches a gentle boil. Cook for another 15 to 20 minutes, covered, with occasional stirring. Cook for 5 more minutes, whisking in the pumpkin and coconut milk.

Fill a blender halfway with soup and process until smooth, working in batches if needed. Before serving, return to a pot and reheat for a few minutes over medium heat.

SALAD WITH BRAISED CARROT

6 Servings | 20 minutes to prepare | 30 minutes to cook | 1 hour and 30 minutes total 295 calories | 23.8 grams of carbohydrates | 19.7 grams of fat | 7.6 grams of protein | 14 milligrams of cholesterol

INGREDIENTS

1 teaspoon honey 1/2 cup slivered almonds 2 pounds peeled and thinly sliced carrots on the diagonal

1 tsp. vinegar

2 garlic cloves, chopped

cranberries, dried, 1/3 cup

extra-virgin olive oil (about 1/4 cup)

1 (4 oz) package crumbled Danish blue cheese salt and pepper to taste

Arugula, 2 cups

DIRECTIONS

Preheat oven to 400 degrees Fahrenheit (200 degrees Celsius) (200 degrees C).

In a large mixing bowl, mix together the carrots, almonds, and garlic. Season to taste with salt and pepper after drizzling with olive oil. Place on a baking sheet that has not been greased.

30 minutes in a preheated oven, bake the carrots until soft and brown on the edges. Allow to cool to room temperature before removing from the oven.

Return the carrots to the mixing bowl once they have cooled, and drizzle with honey and vinegar, tossing to coat. Toss in the cranberries and blue cheese until thoroughly combined. Serve immediately with arugula.

SLOPPY JOES IN TONYA'S WORLD

4 servings | 10 minutes to prepare | 30 minutes to cook 362 calories | 31.2 grams of carbohydrates | 15.3 grams of fat | 23.7 grams of protein | 71 milligrams of cholesterol

INGREDIENTS

2 lb. beef mince

1 1/2 tsp. Worcestershire

1 teaspoon vinegar, 1/2 cup chopped onion

1 celery stalk, chopped

1 teaspoon powdered mustard

ketchup (7 oz.)

lemon juice (1/8 teaspoon)

brown sugar (1 tablespoon)

8 hamburger buns (white or wheat).

DIRECTIONS

Over medium-high heat, place a large skillet. In a large pan, crumble the ground meat; add the onion and celery. Cook, stirring constantly, for 7 to 10 minutes, or until the meat is thoroughly browned.

In a large mixing bowl, combine the meat, ketchup, brown sugar, Worcestershire sauce, vinegar, mustard, and lemon juice. Reduce heat to medium-low and continue to cook, stirring occasionally, until the sauce has thickened and the mixture is heated, approximately 20 minutes.

GRILLED CHEESE SANDWICH WITH A JALAPENO POPPER

2 servings | 10 minutes to prepare | 10 minutes to prepare | 10 minutes to cook | 20 minutes total 528 calories | 40.9

grams of carbohydrates | 34 grams of fat | 16.5 grams of protein | 89 milligrams of cholesterol

INGREDIENTS

softened 2 oz. cream cheese

butter, 4 tsp

sour cream, 1 tblsp

8 crumpled tortilla chips

10 jalapeño pepper slices, chopped, or to taste

1 pound shredded cheese Colby-Monterey Jack is a cheese made by combining the flavors of Colby and Monterey

Sandwich rolls made with ciabatta

DIRECTIONS

In a small mixing bowl, mix together the cream cheese, sour cream, and pickled jalapeo. Remove the item from circulation. Preheat the skillet to medium.

Each roll should be cut in half horizontally, then the rounded tops of the ciabatta rolls should be sliced off to produce a flat top half. 1 teaspoon butter on the doughy cut side of the bottom bun, 1 teaspoon butter on the now-flattened top bun On the unbuttered side of the bottom bun, spread half of the cream cheese mixture, half of the crumbled chips, and half of the shredded cheese. Place the sandwich on the heated pan and top with the remaining half of the bread. Make a second sandwich and repeat the process.

Grill until gently cooked on one side and golden brown on the other, 3 to 5 minutes.

SOUP WITH LEEK AND ROASTED CAULIFLOWER

6 servings | 10 minutes of prep time | 1 hour and 5 minutes of cooking time | 1 hour and 15 minutes total FACTS ABOUT THE NUTRITION

209 calories | 15.4 grams of carbohydrate | 15.9 grams of fat | 3.8 grams of protein | 34 milligrams of cholesterol

INGREDIENTS

2 garlic cloves, chopped

chicken stock (1 quart)

2 tbsp. oil

heavy whipping cream (about a third of a cup)

florets from 1 head of cauliflower

1 tsp chervil (dry)

butter, 3 tablespoons

1 tbsp. salt (kosher)

2 chopped leeks (just the white portion)

1 teaspoon black pepper, freshly cracked

1 tablespoon flour, all-purpose

DIRECTIONS

Preheat the oven to 375°F/190°C/190°C/190°C/190°C (190 degrees C).

In a small bowl, combine garlic and vegetable oil. Place the cauliflower florets on a baking pan and drizzle with the oil mixture. Toss to evenly distribute the ingredients.

30 minutes in a preheated oven, bake cauliflower until soft and gently browned.

Cook and whisk leeks and flour in melted butter in a 4-quart stockpot over medium heat until aromatic and thoroughly mixed, 5 to 10 minutes. Simmer for 20 to 25 minutes, until the cauliflower, chicken stock, and cream have mixed. Stir in the chervil, salt, and pepper, and continue to cook for 10 to 15 minutes longer, or until the soup reaches the desired thickness.

BACON AND BEANS

6 servings | 15 minutes of prep time | 2 hours and 20 minutes of cooking time | 2 hours and 35 minutes of total time FACTS ABOUT THE NUTRITION

631 calories | 52.2 grams of carbs | 35.3 grams of fat | 26.6 grams of protein | 51 milligrams of cholesterol

INGREDIENTS

1 bay leaf 9 cups water 1 (16 ounce) container dry navy beans

1 pound bacon 1 tablespoon salt

black pepper, 1/4 teaspoon

1/8 teaspoon ground garlic cloves 2 chopped onions

1 (16 oz.) container diced tomatoes 2 celery stalks, chopped

4 tsp bouillon de poulet de poulet de poulet de poulet de water (four cups)

DIRECTIONS

Boil the beans for an hour in 9 cups of water. Set aside after draining.

Cook the bacon until it reaches your preferred texture (soft or crisp, as desired), then drain all except 1/4 cup of the fat. The bacon should be coarsely chopped.

In the reserved bacon fat, sauté the onions and celery until tender, but do not drain. Simmer for 2 hours with the chicken stock or cubes, 4 cups water, beans, bay leaf, salt, pepper, and cloves.

Combine the tomatoes and their juice in a large mixing bowl. Serve.

SALAD DE POTATOES

20 servings | 20 minutes to prepare | 10 minutes to cook

FACTS ABOUT THE NUTRITION

339 calories | 20.4 grams of carbs | 27.6 grams of fat | 4.1 grams of protein | 53 milligrams of cholesterol

INGREDIENTS

5 lb. chopped red potatoes

1 celery stalk, chopped

mayonnaise (three cups)

3 tsp mustard (prepared)

2 c. pickled cucumbers, coarsely chopped

1 TBS ACV

1 teaspoon salt (or to taste) 5 hard-boiled eggs, diced

1 red onion, chopped

1 teaspoon black pepper, freshly ground

DIRECTIONS

Bring salted water to a boil over potatoes in a big saucepan. Reduce the heat to mediumlow and continue to cook for another 10 minutes, or until the vegetables are soft. Drain. While the dressing is being made, return the potatoes to the empty saucepan to dry. salt

In a large mixing bowl, combine the mayonnaise, pickles, hard-boiled eggs, red onion, celery, mustard, cider vinegar, 1 teaspoon salt, and pepper. In a large mixing bowl, combine the potatoes and mayonnaise. Before serving, refrigerate the dish for at least six hours or overnight.

SHRIMP OF CAJUN

4 servings | 5 minutes to prepare | 5 minutes to prepare | 5 minutes to cook | 10 minutes total FACTS ABOUT THE NUTRITION

166 calories | 0.9 grams of carbohydrate | 5 grams of fat | 28 grams of protein | 259 milligrams of cholesterol

INGREDIENTS

paprika, 1 tblsp.

black pepper, 1/4 teaspoon

dried thyme, 3/4 teaspoon

cayenne pepper, 1/4 teaspoon (or more to taste)

1 tsp. oregano (dried)

peeled and deveined 1 1/2 pounds big shrimp

garlic powder, 1/4 teaspoon

1 tsp. oil

salt (quarter teaspoon)

DIRECTIONS

In a sealable plastic bag, mix together the paprika, thyme, oregano, garlic powder, salt, pepper, and cayenne pepper. Shake to coat shrimp.

In a large nonstick skillet, heat the oil on medium high. Cook and stir shrimp in hot oil for approximately 4 minutes, or until they are brilliant pink on the exterior and the flesh is no longer translucent in the middle.

POTATO SOUP WITH MANDI'S CHEESE

5 people | 10 minutes to prepare | 35 minutes to cook | 45 minutes total FACTS ABOUT THE NUTRITION

466 calories | 51 grams of carbs | 21.5 grams of fat | 18.7 grams of protein | 45 milligrams of cholesterol

INGREDIENTS

3 tablespoons margarine, melted 5 peeled and diced potatoes

1 finely sliced carrot

all-purpose flour, 3 tblsp

finely sliced celery stalk

steak seasoning (1 1/2 teaspoons)

1 teaspoon black pepper 1 1/2 cup water

1 tsp sodium

2 cups four-cheese shredded mixture

milk, 2 1/2 c.

DIRECTIONS

Toss potatoes, carrots, celery, water, and salt in a large saucepan over medium heat. Bring to a boil, then lower to a low heat, cover, and cook for 15 to 20 minutes, until the potatoes are cooked. Stir in the milk when the vegetables are soft.

Melted margarine, flour, steak seasoning, and pepper should all be combined in a small basin. Stir into the soup, then boil, stirring constantly, until thick and bubbling. Remove the pan from the heat and toss in the cheese until it is completely melted. Before serving, set aside for 5 to 10 minutes.

FRIED RICE WITH THAI SPICY BASIL CHICKEN

6 servings | 30 minutes of prep time | 10 minutes of cooking time | 40 minutes total 794 calories | 116.4 grams of carbohydrates | 22.1 grams of fat | 29.1 grams of protein | 46 milligrams of cholesterol

INGREDIENTS

oyster sauce (3 tablespoons)

1 pound chicken breast, boneless and skinless, cut into thin strips

2 tsp. soy sauce

1 finely sliced and seeded red pepper

1 tsp. sugar

1 finely sliced onion (about 1 cup)

frying oil: 1/2 cup peanut

2 c Thai basil, sweet

4 cups cooked and cooled jasmine rice

1 slice of cucumber (optional)

garlic cloves, smashed, 6 big cloves

cilantro sprigs (half a cup) (optional)

crushed serrano peppers

DIRECTIONS

In a large mixing basin, combine the oyster sauce, fish sauce, and sugar.

In a wok, heat the oil until it starts to smoke over medium-high heat. Stir rapidly to incorporate the garlic and serrano peppers. Cook, stirring constantly, until the chicken is no longer pink, adding the bell pepper, onion, and oyster sauce combination. Raise the heat to high and immediately whisk in the cold rice, making sure the sauce is well combined. Break apart any rice that's stuck together using the back of a spoon.

Take the pan off the heat and add the basil leaves. As desired, garnish with cucumber slices and cilantro.

SMOKED SAUSAGE WITH CABBAGE PASTA

6 people | 15 minutes to prepare | 20 minutes to cook | 35 minutes total 845 calories | 68.5 grams of carbohydrate | 51.2 grams of fat | 30.9 grams of protein | 95 milligrams of cholesterol

INGREDIENTS

1 farfalle (bow tie) pasta (16 ounce package)

1 big shredded head of green cabbage

1 tablespoon of butter

to taste with salt and pepper

2 garlic cloves, chopped

1 pound thinly sliced smoked sausage

olive oil, 1/4 cup

Parmesan cheese (grated): 1/4 cup

DIRECTIONS

Bring a big saucepan of lightly salted water to a boil over high heat. Stir in the bow tie spaghetti and bring to a boil once the water has reached a boil. Cook, uncovered, for approximately 12 minutes, or until the pasta is cooked through but still firm to the biting. Drain well in a sink colander.

In a big saucepan over medium heat, melt the butter. Season with salt and pepper, then add the garlic, olive oil, and cabbage. Cook for 15 minutes, or until the cabbage is soft. Cook for another 5 minutes, or until the sausage and bow tie pasta are fully warm. Serve immediately, topped with Parmesan cheese.

BUTTERNUT SQUASH SOUP WITH CARAMELIZED BUTTERNUT

12 people | 20 minutes to prepare | 30 minutes to cook | 50 minutes total Calories: 189 | Carbohydrates: 24.9g | Fat: 10.3g | Protein: 2.9g | Cholesterol: 23mg NUTRITION FACTS Calories: 189 | Carbohydrates: 24.9g | Fat: 10.3g | Protein: 2.9g

INGREDIENTS

extra-virgin olive oil, 3 tblsp.

4 cup chicken broth (or more if necessary)

1/4 cup honey 3 pounds peeled and diced butternut squash

1 chopped big onion

heavy whipping cream (1/2 cup)

butter, 3 tablespoons

1 tsp. nutmeg powder, or to taste

1 tbsp. salt (to taste)

1 teaspoon white pepper, freshly cracked, to taste

DIRECTIONS

In a big saucepan over high heat, heat olive oil. In a heated skillet, cook and stir squash for approximately 10 minutes, or until it is thoroughly browned. Cook and toss the squash with the onion, butter, sea salt, and cracked white pepper for approximately 10 minutes, or until the onions are totally soft and starting to brown.

Bring the chicken stock and honey to a boil over the squash, then lower to a low heat and cook for 5 minutes, or until the squash is soft.

Fill a blender just halfway with the mixture. Cover and secure the lid, then pulse a few times to combine. Until smooth, puree in batches.

To serve, whisk together the cream, nutmeg, salt, and freshly ground white pepper.

TOMATO SOUP WITH ROASTED INGREDIENTS

NUTRITION FACTS: 6 SERVINGS | 10 MINUTES TO PREPARE | 50 MINUTES TO COOK

140 calories | 14.7 grams of carbs | 7.6 grams of fat | 5.4 grams of protein | 3 milligrams of cholesterol

INGREDIENTS

1 1/2 teaspoon freshly ground black pepper 3 pounds roma (plum) tomatoes, quartered

1 half-and-quartered yellow onion

3 garlic cloves, quartered

5 cups chicken broth (low sodium) 1/2 red bell pepper, diced olive oil, 3 tablespoons

2 tsp. basil powder

a pinch of salt

1 tsp parsley, dry

DIRECTIONS

Preheat the oven to 400 degrees Fahrenheit (200 degrees Celsius) (200 degrees C). Wrap aluminum foil around a large baking sheet.

On the prepared baking sheet, arrange the tomatoes, onion, and red bell pepper in one layer. Season with salt and pepper and drizzle olive oil over tomato mixture.

Cook for 30 minutes in a preheated oven; add the garlic and roast for another 15 minutes, or until the tomato mixture is soft.

In a large stockpot, bring the chicken broth, basil, and parsley to a boil; decrease heat to low and continue to cook.

In a blender, puree half of the tomato sauce. Cover and let aside; pulse a few times before blending until smooth, adding a tiny amount of heated chicken broth if necessary. Fill a stockpot halfway with chicken broth and purée the tomato mixture. Half of the tomato combination should be pureed and added to the chicken stock mixture. 5 minutes on low heat

MELT IN THE CALIFORNIA

4 servings | 15 minutes to prepare | 2 minutes to cook FACTS ABOUT THE NUTRITION

335 calories | 21.1 grams of carbs | 22.5 grams of fat | 15.6 grams of protein | 26 milligrams of cholesterol

INGREDIENTS

4 pieces gently toasted wholegrain bread

toasted almonds, 1/3 cup

1 cup sliced mushrooms 1 avocado (sliced) 1 tomato (sliced)

Swiss cheese, 4 pieces

DIRECTIONS

Preheat the broiler on high in the oven.

On a baking pan, place the toasted bread. 1/4 avocado, mushrooms, almonds, and tomato slices are spread on each piece of bread. A piece of Swiss cheese should be placed on top of each.

Broil the open-face sandwiches for approximately 2 minutes, or until the cheese starts to melt and bubble. Warm sandwiches should be served.

VERY EASY AND QUICK DUMPLINGS WITH CHICKEN

6 people | 5 minutes to prepare | 15 minutes to cook | 20 minutes total FACTS ABOUT THE NUTRITION

361 calories | 29.6 grams of carbs | 15.1 grams of fat | 25 grams of protein | 63 milligrams of cholesterol

INGREDIENTS

2 14 cup baking powder

2/3 cup milk 2 cans (14 ounce) chicken broth

2 drained chunk chicken cans (10 ounces)

DIRECTIONS

Combine the biscuit mix and milk in a medium mixing dish and whisk until combined. Remove the item from circulation.

Bring the chicken broth and the cans of chicken broth to a boil in a saucepan together. Take a handful of biscuit dough and flatten it in your hands after the broth has reached a steady boil. Cut 1 to 2 inch pieces and place them into the simmering soup. At the very least, make sure they are completely submerged. When all of the dough has been added to the saucepan, gently stir to ensure that the broth covers the newest dough clumps. Cover and cook, stirring periodically, for 10 minutes over medium heat.

BURGERS WITH VEGAN BLACK BEAN

4 servings | 15 minutes to prepare | 20 minutes to prepare | 35 minutes total FACTS ABOUT THE NUTRITION

264 calories | 51.7 grams of carbs | 1.4 grams of fat | 11.6 grams of protein | 0 milligrams of cholesterol

INGREDIENTS

1 can (15 ounces) drained and rinsed black beans

1 tsp cayenne

1 cup sweet onion, chopped

cumin powder (1 teaspoon)

garlic, minced 1 tablespoon

1 tsp. sea salt (such as Old Bay)

3 peeled and shredded baby carrots (optional)

salt (quarter teaspoon)

green bell pepper, minced 1/4 cup (optional)

black pepper, 1/4 teaspoon

cornstarch (1 tablespoon)

2 slices whole-wheat bread, shredded

1 tsp. water

a third of a cup of unbleached flour, or more if required

3 tablespoons chile-garlic sauce (Sriracha, for example), or to taste

DIRECTIONS

Preheat the oven to 350 degrees Fahrenheit (180 degrees Celsius) (175 degrees C). Preheat the oven to 350°F. Prepare a baking sheet by greasing it.

In a mixing basin, combine the black beans, onion, garlic, carrots, and green bell pepper; mash well. Mix.

In a separate small mixing bowl, combine cornstarch, water, chile-garlic sauce, chili powder, cumin, seafood seasoning, salt, and black pepper. In a separate bowl, whisk together the cornstarch and water. Add the cornstarch mixture to the black bean mixture and

Combine the beans with the whole-wheat bread. 1/4 cup flour at a time, until a sticky batter develops, stir flour into bean mixture.

Using a 3/4-inch thickness per mound, spoon burger-sized mounds of batter onto the prepared baking sheet. To make burgers, combine all of the ingredients in a bowl and form into

Cook for approximately 10 minutes on each side in a preheated oven until the center is done and the exterior is crisp.

SOUP WITH ASPARAGUS CREAM AND MUSSELS

8 people | 15 minutes to prepare | 40 minutes to cook | 55 minutes total FACTS ABOUT THE NUTRITION

171 calories | 12.7 grams of carbs | 11.8 grams of fat | 5.2 grams of protein | 29 milligrams of cholesterol

INGREDIENTS

3 bacon slivers

1 tablespoon bacon drippings (6 cups chicken broth) peeled and diced 1 potato

1 teaspoon of butter

1 pound asparagus spears, tips and stalks set aside chopped

3 celery stalks, salt and pepper to taste

1 chopped onion

8 oz. fresh mushrooms, sliced

all-purpose flour, 3 tblsp

a third of a cup of half-and-half

DIRECTIONS

Cook, turning occasionally, until evenly browned, about 10 minutes, in a large, deep skillet over medium-high heat. On a paper towel–lined plate, drain the bacon slices. When the bacon is cool enough to handle, crumble it and place it aside. 1 tablespoon bacon drippings should be kept aside.

In a saucepan over medium heat, melt butter and drippings.

In a large saucepan, cook and stir celery and onion for 4 minutes, or until onion is translucent.

Cook for 1 minute while whisking in the flour.

Bring to a boil, whisking in chicken broth.

Reserving the asparagus tips for later, add the potato and chopped asparagus stalks. Salt and black pepper to taste.

Simmer for 20 minutes after lowering the heat.

Fill a blender halfway with soup. Using a folded kitchen towel to hold down the lid of the blender, carefully start it, using a few quick pulses to get the soup moving before leaving it on to puree. In a clean pot, puree in batches until smooth. You can also puree the soup in the cooking pot with a stick blender.

In the same skillet as the bacon, cook and stir mushrooms and asparagus tips until liquid has evaporated, about 5 to 8 minutes. If necessary, season with salt and pepper.

To make the pureed soup, add the mushrooms, asparagus tips, and half-and-half cream. Cook until everything is completely warm.

Crumbled bacon can be used to garnish the soup.

SLOW-COOKER CHILI WITH VEGAN INGREDIENTS

15 servings | 45 minutes of preparation time | 5 hours and 10 minutes of cooking time | 5 hours and 55 minutes of total time Calories: 134 | Carbohydrates: 24.8g | Fat: 2.4g |

Protein: 6.3g | Cholesterol: 0mg NUTRITION FACTS Calories: 134 | Carbohydrates: 24.8g | Fat: 2.4g | Protein: 6.3g

INGREDIENTS

1 teaspoon of extra virgin olive oil

1 tbsp. oregano (dried)

1 finely chopped green bell pepper

1 tsp parsley powder

1/2 teaspoon salt, 1 red bell pepper, chopped

1/2 teaspoon ground black pepper 1 yellow bell pepper (chopped)

2 chopped onions 2 diced tomatoes with juice (14.5 oz.)

1 (15 oz) can black beans, rinsed and drained 4 garlic cloves, minced

1 cup frozen corn kernels, thawed 1 (15 ounce) can kidney beans, rinsed and drained 1 (10 ounce) package frozen chopped spinach, thawed and drained

2 (6 oz.) cans tomato paste 1 zucchini, chopped

1 (8-ounce) can tomato sauce (or more if needed) 1 yellow squash, chopped

chili powder, 6 tbsp

1 cup vegetable broth, plus a little extra if necessary

cumin powder (1 tablespoon)

DIRECTIONS

Cook the green, red, and yellow bell peppers, onions, and garlic in olive oil in a large skillet over medium heat for 8 to 10 minutes, or until the onions begin to brown. In a slow cooker, place the mixture. Toss in the spinach, corn, zucchini, yellow squash, chili powder, cumin, oregano, parsley, salt, black pepper, tomatoes, black beans, garbanzo beans, kidney beans, and tomato paste until everything is well combined. Toss the ingredients with the tomato sauce and vegetable broth.

Cook on low for 4 to 5 hours, or until all of the vegetables are tender. Check for seasoning; if the chili is too thick, add more tomato sauce and vegetable broth until it reaches the desired consistency. To blend the flavors, cook for an additional 1 to 2 hours.

SALAD WITH QUINOA AND VEGANS

12 servings | 20 minutes of prep time | 25 minutes of cooking time | 1 hour and 30 minutes of total time FACTS ABOUT THE NUTRITION

148 calories | 22.9 grams of carbohydrate | 4.5 grams of fat | 4.6 grams of protein | 0 milligrams of cholesterol

INGREDIENTS

1 tsp. oil from canola

half a cucumber, diced

garlic, minced 1 tablespoon

thawed corn kernels, 1/2 cup

a quarter cup chopped (yellow or purple) onion

red onion, diced

1 1/2 tablespoons fresh chopped cilantro 2 1/2 cups water

1 tablespoon chopped fresh mint 2 teaspoons salt (or to taste)

black pepper, 1/4 teaspoon

1 tsp sodium

quinoa, 2 cup

black pepper, 1/4 teaspoon

fresh tomato, diced

olive oil, 2 tablespoons

carrots, 3/4 cup diced

balsamic vinegar, 3 tablespoons

yellow bell pepper, diced

DIRECTIONS

In a saucepan on medium heat, heat the canola oil. 5 minutes in the hot oil, cook and stir the garlic and 1/4 cup onion until the onion softens and turns translucent. Bring the water, 2 teaspoons salt, and 1/4 teaspoon black pepper to a boil, then add the quinoa and cover. Cook for about 20 minutes, or until quinoa is tender. Transfer the quinoa to a large mixing bowl after draining any remaining water with a mesh strainer. Allow to cool before serving.

In a chilled quinoa bowl, mix together the tomato, carrots, bell pepper, cucumber, corn, and 1/4 cup red onion. 1 teaspoon salt, 1/4 teaspoon black pepper, cilantro, mint, 1 teaspoon salt Pour the olive oil and balsamic vinegar over the salad and toss gently to combine.

RESTAURANT-STYLE ITALIAN SUBSCRIPTIONS

8 servings | 20 minutes to prepare | 1 hour to cook | 1 hour and 20 minutes total FACTS ABOUT THE NUTRITION

708 calories | 40.4 grams of carbs | 47.3 grams of fat | 29.2 grams of protein | 79 milligrams of cholesterol

INGREDIENTS

1 rinsed and torn head red leaf lettuce

red pepper flakes (1/4 teaspoon)

2 c. chopped fresh tomatoes

1 tsp oregano (dried)

1 finely chopped medium red onion

Capacola sausage, sliced, 1/2 pound

olive oil (six tablespoons)

Genoa salami, 1/2 pound thinly sliced

white wine vinegar, 2 tblsp

2 tablespoons fresh parsley, chopped 1/4 pound thinly sliced prosciutto

Provolone cheese, sliced, 1/2 pound

4 submarine rolls, split 2 garlic cloves (chopped)

1 tsp basil powder

1 cup slices of dill pickle

DIRECTIONS

Combine the lettuce, tomatoes, and onion in a large mixing bowl. Combine the olive oil, white wine vinegar, parsley, garlic, basil, red pepper flakes, and oregano in a separate bowl and whisk to combine. Toss the salad to evenly coat it with the dressing. 1 hour in the refrigerator

Layer the Capacola, salami, prosciutto, and provolone cheese evenly on each submarine roll. Add some salad and as many pickle slices as you'd like. Close and serve the rolls.

JIM'S ONION SODA WITH CHEDDAR BREAD

12 people | 15 minutes to prepare | 30 minutes to cook | 55 minutes total FACTS ABOUT THE NUTRITION

264 calories | 36.9 grams of carbs | 9.1 grams of fat | 8.2 grams of protein | 24 milligrams of cholesterol

INGREDIENTS

1 1/4 cup buttermilk 4 cups bread flour + more for dusting

2 tbsp. confectioners' sugar 1 1/2 tsp. salt

1 tbsp flour

onion, finely chopped (approximately 3/4 cup)

6 tbsp. softened butter

Cheddar cheese, shredded

DIRECTIONS

Preheat the oven to 425 degrees Fahrenheit (200 degrees Celsius) (220 degrees C). Use parchment paper to cover a baking sheet.

Combine bread flour, salt, and baking powder in a large mixing bowl and whisk until well combined. To make a dough, combine the butter, buttermilk, and confectioners' sugar; add the onion and Cheddar cheese and gently combine. Make two balls out of the dough by dividing it in half. Flatten the loaves to about 2 inches thick on the prepared baking sheet. Make a flour dusting on each loaf.

Preheat the oven to 350°F and bake for 30 minutes, or until golden brown. Cool for a few minutes on wire racks before serving.